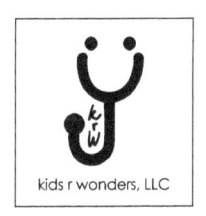

# The KIDS' MEDICAL CARE HANDBOOK

Kathie R. Wuellner, MD, FAAP

kids r wonders, LLC

Copyright ©2025 by Kathie R. Wuellner

All rights reserved.

No part of this publication may be reproduced or transmitted in any form or by any means, electronic or mechanical, including photography, recording, or any information storage and retrieval system, without permission in writing from the author.

Requests for permission to make copies of any part of the work should be emailed to the following address: drkathie@kidsrwonders.com.
The advice and strategies contained herein may not be suitable for your situation. The publisher and the author make no guarantee of the results obtained by using this book.
Neither the publisher nor the author shall be liable for any damages.

Published and distributed by Kids R Wonders, LLC
Alton, USA

Wuellner, Kathie
The Kids' Medical Care Handbook
ISBN 979-8-9918202-0-2 Paperback

# CONTENTS

1. The **HEAD** .................... 9
2. The **EAR** ..................... 23
3. The **EYE** ..................... 33
4. The **NOSE** .................... 39
5. The **THROAT** .................. 47
6. The **CHEST** ................... 57
7. The **HEART** ................... 77
8. The **ABDOMEN** ................. 85
9. The **GENITO URINARY SYSTEM** .......... 115
10. The **EXTREMITIES** ............ 135
11. The **SKIN** ................... 149

**MISCELLANEOUS** .................. 213
**FIRST AID** ...................... 227
**APPENDIX** ....................... 233
**INDEX** .......................... 247

# INTRODUCTION

Have you ever been up in the middle of the night, worrying about your sick infant or child? Have you been on vacation and your child developed a rash, leaving you unsure of what it was or what to do for it? Have you ever debated whether to call your child's provider with a question about your child, only to regret not doing so when the problem worsened after the provider's office closed for the day?

I have compiled this book with notes and pictures to help you through these situations and much more. The purpose of this book is to:

- Provide immediate advice for parents and caregivers of children.
- Help parents and caregivers understand various medical conditions that children experience.
- Empower parents and caregivers to make informed decisions about their children's health

As a practicing private pediatrician and a parent for over 40 years, I would like to share the following observations and experiences:

- Parenting is not easy, especially for first-time parents.
- Parenting is stressful.
- Caring for a sick child, whether in the middle of the night or during the day, can be overwhelming.
- Children do not come with instruction manuals.
- Children are not "little adults" and should not be medically managed as such.
- There is not always enough time during a child's office visit to discuss all pertinent information. Additionally, in the moment, the parent with a sick child may not have enough mental energy to ask more questions. There may also be distractions during the office visit – for example, your child cries throughout the entire visit.

This book aims to help parents and caregivers understand what goes on in medical conditions that children experience. I hope to offer information that reduces the need to visit Urgent Cares and Emergency Rooms because of fear and uncertainty when the pediatric provider is not available. Urgent Cares and Emergency Rooms are not normally staffed with providers specifically and extensively trained in pediatrics (except for Pediatric Urgent Care facilities or Pediatric Emergency Rooms). The importance of using your child's pediatric provider for all their medical needs is stressed, as the provider is the source of all-encompassing information about your child.

I also wanted to provide "standard-of-care", tried and proven information and advice for parents to use. This includes guidance on what can be done at home, when to call the child's healtchcare provider, or when to seek emergency medical assistance.

Lastly, don't forget to hug your child(ren) today!
Hugs are the best medicine!

Kathie R. Wuellner, MD, FAAP

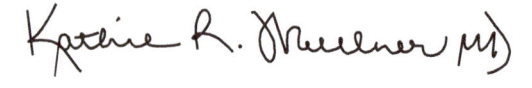

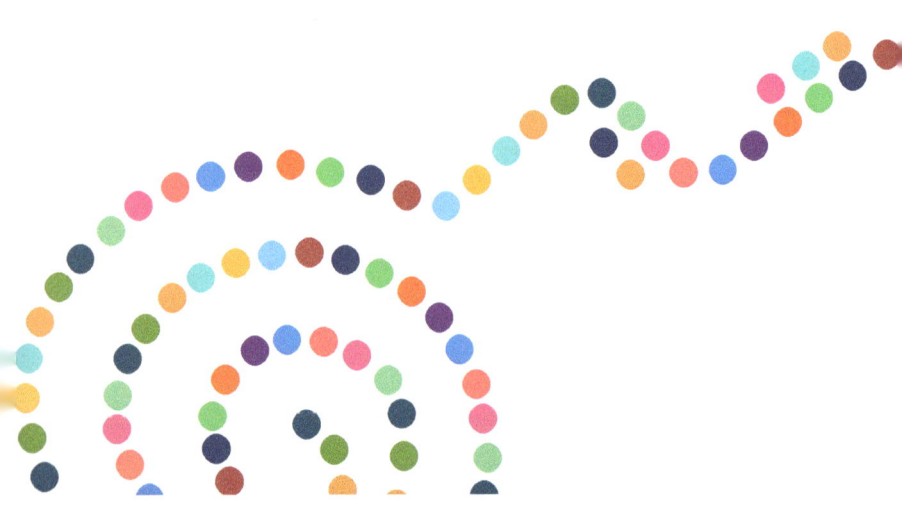

## Useful Lists 7

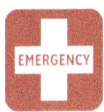

### CALL 911
### In any life-threatening emergeny.

**Have the following information ready:**

- **LOCATION OF EMERGENCY.**
- **PHONE NUMBER YOU ARE CALLING FROM.**
- **NATURE OF EMERGENCY.**
- **DETAILS ABOUT EMERGENCY**

# EMERGENCY CONTACTS:

- **POISON CONTROL: 800-222-1222**
- **POLICE DEPARTMENT:** ........................................................................
- **FIRE DEPARTMENT:** ...........................................................................

- **DOCTOR:**

    Name: ........................................................................................................
    Number: ....................................................................................................

- **DENTIST:**

    Name: ........................................................................................................
    Number: ....................................................................................................

- **FAMILY, FRIENDS, NEIGHBORS:**

    - Name/relationship: ..............................................................................
      Number: ................................................................................................

    - Name/relationship: ..............................................................................
      Number: ................................................................................................

    - Name/relationship: ..............................................................................
      Number: ................................................................................................

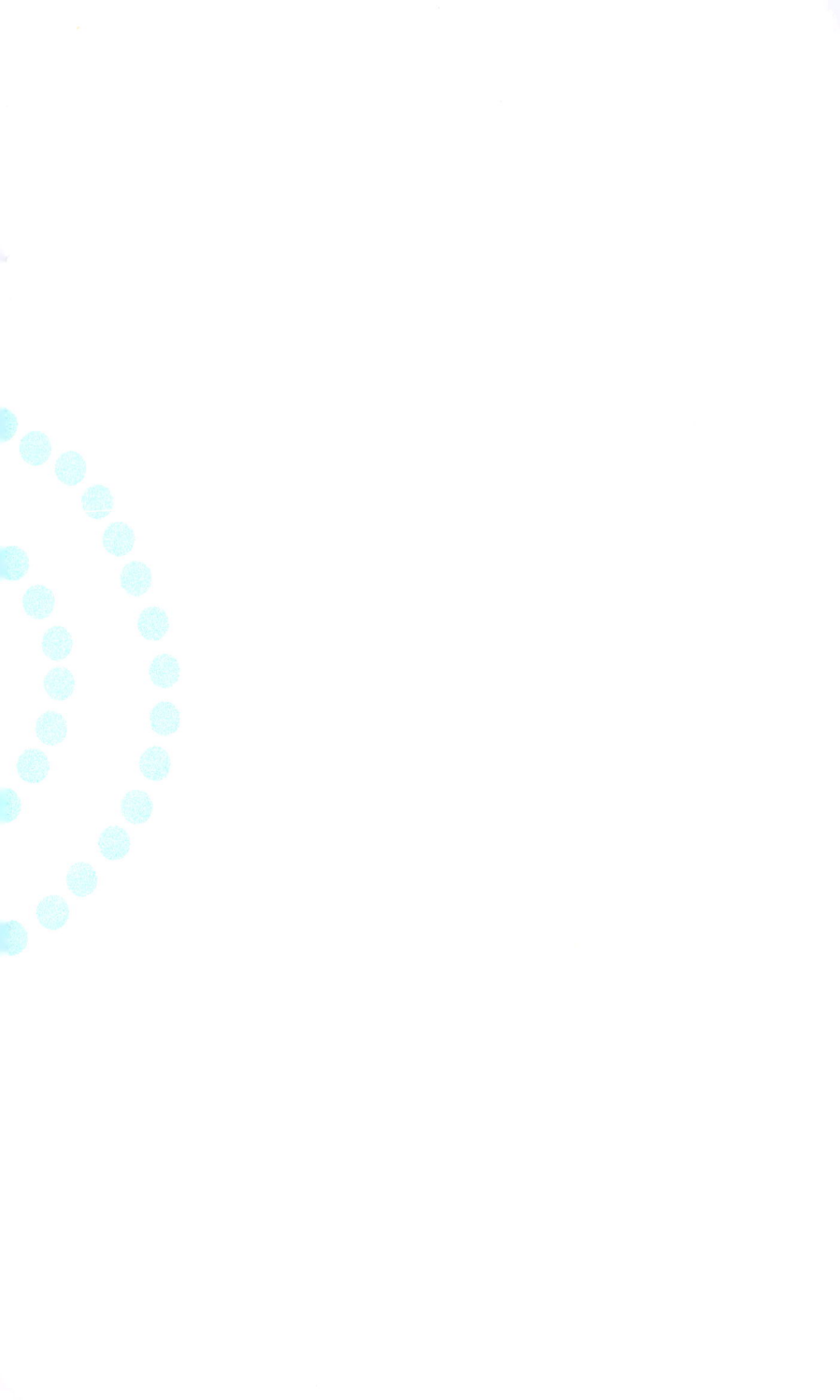

# CHAPTER 1
# THE HEAD

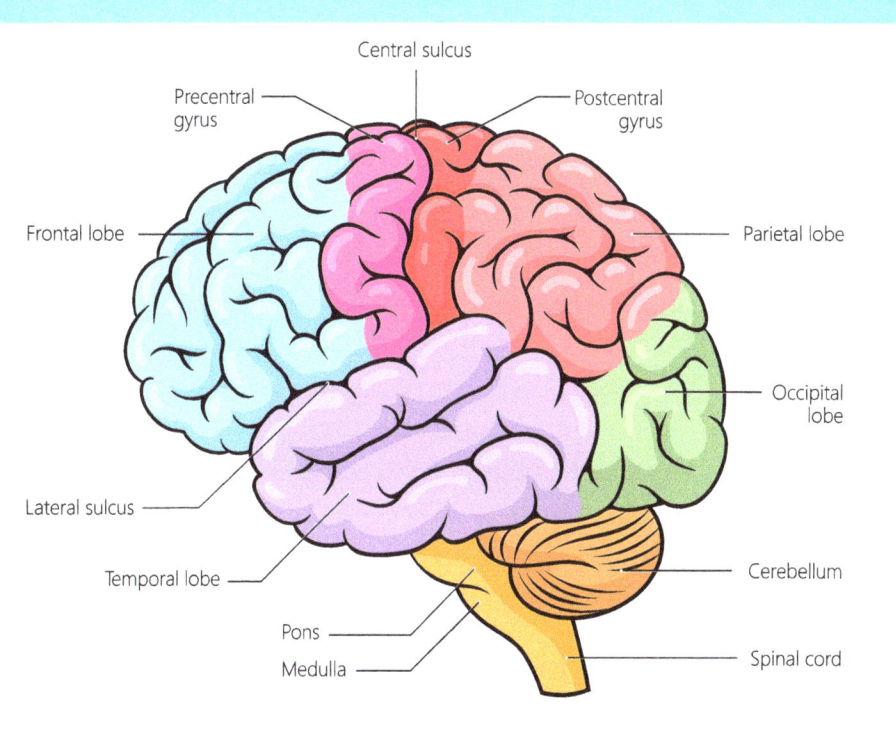

- Central sulcus
- Precentral gyrus
- Postcentral gyrus
- Frontal lobe
- Parietal lobe
- Occipital lobe
- Lateral sulcus
- Temporal lobe
- Cerebellum
- Pons
- Medulla
- Spinal cord

Alexander_P/Shutterstock

## 10 The Head

# HEAD TRAUMA:

Head trauma in children occurs fairly frequently. All children are "careless" to a certain extent and toddlers "know no fear". There are different methods of how the head is injured, but we divide injuries into two groups: MINOR and MAJOR HEAD TRAUMA.

## CAUSES:

MINOR HEAD TRAUMA:
- Occurs from falls of short heights (under 4 feet), toddlers running into walls, tripping, and falling onto the ground, striking the head.

MAJOR HEAD TRAUMA:
- May occur from falls of higher distances (greater than 5 feet), colliding with another person while running, motor vehicle accidents, bicycle accidents, and all-terrain vehicle accidents, to name a few.

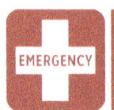

### WHEN TO CALL 911 or GO TO THE EMERGENCY ROOM

- **The child is unconscious.**
- **There is more than one episode of vomiting.**
- **Child is unable to stay awake.**
- **Child is having a seizure.**
- **Child is having bloody or clear drainage coming from ear.**
- **Child has unequal pupil size.**

**DO NOT MOVE AN UNCONSCIOUS CHILD** (unless the location is more dangerous than moving the child). If you do have to move the child, make every effort to stabilize the neck in case of concurrent neck injury.

## WHAT TO DO AT HOME:

- In the event of minor head trauma (child cried immediately, is alert, crying, moving all extremities), and if none of the alarming symptoms previously described develop, it is appropriate to watch the child at home.
- In minor head trauma, the child may develop a "goose egg" which is bleeding underneath the skin but on the outside of the skull. An ice bag will help minimize the swelling/bruising if your child will let you place one; it is not absolutely necessary to treat with an ice bag.
- In the situation of minor head trauma, try to keep your child more quiet for the next 24 hours following the head trauma to help in recovery.

## HOW TO PREVENT HEAD INJURIES:

- Reduce hazards around the house that could allow children to hurt themselves.
- Install safety gates in front of stairs, minimize throw rugs on floors.
- Insist that your child always wears a helmet when riding a bike or scooter.
- Ensure that your child is properly harnessed into a car seat or booster seat while riding in a vehicle. Do not forget your own seat belt!
- Insist that your child always wears a helmet when riding an all-terrain vehicle.

## SCALP LACERATIONS FROM MINOR HEAD TRAUMA:

### CAUSES:
- Common in toddlers and younger children, who fall often.

### SYMPTOMS:
- Usually very superficial and in a straight line.
- Bleed easily (but total amount of blood is not much).

### WHAT TO DO AT HOME:
- When your child falls and suffers a head injury, always make sure that your child is awake and alert, speaking normally, and moving all extremities. If all of these are working, then the primary focus can be on the laceration.
- **If your child is not alert, not speaking normally, is having a seizure, or is otherwise not acting normally, call 911 or go to your nearest emergency room.**
- Be calm and help your child relax.
- Using a clean rag, tissue, or gauze, apply pressure to the wound. This should stop the bleeding.
- Once the bleeding has stopped, it will be easier to look at the wound and estimate the length of it.

    #### IF THE LACERATION IS LESS THAN 1/2 INCH LONG:
    - It would be better for the child to have it "butterflied" by you at home.
    To "butterfly", simply cut a band aid down to a size that you can use to cover the laceration in a perpendicular fashion. Place the band aid down on one side of the laceration, then pull it over the laceration to line up the edges of the laceration and then place the other end down on the skin on the opposite side of the laceration.

## The Head 13

### WHEN TO CONTACT YOUR CHILD'S HEALTHCARE PROVIDER

- **When the laceration is closer to 1 inch long.**

**IF THE LACERATION IS CLOSE TO 1 INCH OR LONGER:**

- Having sutures placed or having the laceration "glued" would be recommended. Contact your child's physician to obtain recommendations as to where to go for this. An Emergency Room would be able to provide this service.

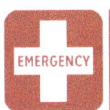

### WHEN TO CALL 911 or GO TO THE EMERGENCY ROOM

- **When your child is not alert, not speaking normally or having a seizure.**

## IMPORTANT:

- **After the laceration has been repaired:**
- Keep the laceration dry for at least 5 days, avoiding getting the area wet with bathing or hair shampooing.
- Scalp lacerations heal fairly quickly. If sutures or staples are used, they can be removed in 5 days.

# HEADACHES:

> Headaches in children are usually not from a serious cause.

## CAUSES:

- A minor illness.
- Bump to the head.
- Lack of sleep.
- Not having had enough to eat or drink in the previous 12-24 hours.
- Stress.
- Becoming overheated.
- Noisy surroundings.

## TYPES:

- **MIGRAINES**
- **MUSCLE TENSION (OR STRESS TYPE)**
- There are other less common types of headaches in children. They are seen infrequently and will not be covered in this book.

# MIGRAINE HEADACHES:

> Can occur in infants as well as older children. May occur infrequently or several times a week. Sometimes there is a family history of migraine headaches.

## SYMPTOMS:

- Usually, there is an acute onset of headache followed by vomiting or nausea; usually after vomiting, the child will fall asleep and sleep for a few hours and then wake up feeling better.

# The Head 15

- Child may have extreme light or hearing sensitivity during the headache.
- Headache is usually pulsating and on one side.

## WHAT TO DO AT HOME:

- If any of the above symptoms are present, give a dose of ibuprofen as soon as possible (see dosage chart in appendix).
- Some children will need medication for vomiting as well.
- Place the child in a dark, quiet room and encourage rest.

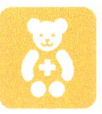

### WHEN TO CONTACT YOUR CHILD'S HEALTHCARE PROVIDER

- **If your child has symptoms of a migraine headache, it is important for the diagnosis to be confirmed by your child's medical provider. Recommendations for treating future headaches will be discussed and medications may be recommended.**
- **If there are repeated migraine headaches despite treatment.**

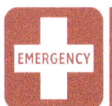

### WHEN TO CALL 911 or GO TO THE EMERGENCY ROOM

- **When your child has an uncontrollable headache despite treatment.**

## MUSCLE TENSION (STRESS) HEADACHES:

> Fairly common type in children.

### SYMPTOMS:
- Tightness of muscles of the head and/or neck.
- Non-pulsating pain on sides or top of the head.
- No vomiting or nausea are present.
- Headache not made worse by physical activity.

### WHAT TO DO AT HOME:
- Give your child a healthy snack and drink (milk or water).
- Have your child rest in a quiet, darkened room and massage the location of your child's headache.
- Do not give a pain reliever (acetaminophen or ibuprofen) unless the headache does not go away after one hour.

### IMPORTANT:
- It is not recommended to give pain relievers with each and every tension headache; too frequent (daily) administration of pain relievers can lead to "rebound headaches".

### WHEN TO CONTACT YOUR CHILD'S HEALTHCARE PROVIDER
- **The headache wakes the child up from sleep.**
- **There is fever and neck rigidity.**
- **There is persistent vomiting or vision changes.**
- **The headaches occur after head trauma.**
- **If tension headaches start to occur several times a week.**

# SEIZURES (CONVULSIONS):

Certain brain cells get "excited" and fire off more rapidly than what they are supposed to; this then disrupts the normal brain electrical activity and leads to the abnormal movements that occur during a seizure. Seizures are fairly common in infants and younger children.

## CAUSES IN CHILDREN:
- Often, a cause of the seizure cannot be determined.
- Fever (the seizure is not triggered by the high degree of the body temperature at that time, but rather how quickly the body temperature rises over a short period of time).
- Head injury.
- Positive family history of seizures.
- Congenital conditions.
- Some poisonings.
- Meningitis.
- Brain tumor.

## SYMPTOMS OR SIGNS OF A SEIZURE :
- Jerking or convulsions of arms and legs.
- Staring.
- Stiffness of the body.
- Loss of consciousness.
- Loss of urine or stool in the presence of other listed symptoms.
- Falling or collapsing suddenly.
- Confusion.
- Rapid eye blinking.

## WHAT TO DO AT HOME:

- Lay the child on the floor or other flat surface.
- Lay the child on his/her right side to minimize aspiration in case of vomiting.
- Remove any objects close by that the child may hit during the seizure.
- Make sure that breathing remains close to normal; check the position of the head and neck to make sure that the airway is open.
- Stay with the child while the seizure is present.
- Call 911 if the seizure lasts more than 5 minutes.
- If possible, try to pay as much attention as you can to the seizure:

    - What part of the body it started in.
    - The length of time of the seizure.
    - What kind of movements were present.
    - What the child was doing right before the seizure.

### WHEN TO CONTACT YOUR CHILD'S HEALTHCARE PROVIDER

- **Once the seizure has stopped.**
- **If it is your child's first seizure, call your child's provider immediately to obtain recommendations for timely evaluation.**
- **If it is not your child's first seizure, call your child's provider or seizure specialist if he/she has one for further instructions. Often times, pediatric neurologists will develop a seizure action plan (instructions to follow in case of a seizure) for patients with known seizures.**

## The Head     19

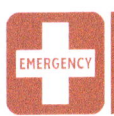

> **WHEN TO CALL 911 or GO TO THE EMERGENCY ROOM**
>
> ▸ **If this is the child's first seizure, and you are unable to contact your provider for directions, take your child to the Emergency Room or call 911.**
>
> ▸ **If the seizure lasts for more than 5 minutes (regardless if it is a first seizure or not) – call 911.**

## DIAGNOSIS AND TREATMENT:

- Much of the work up of a new seizure is based upon what else has been recently going on with the child.
- Tests that are often done (but not necessary in every case) include:
    - Blood tests – CBC. Blood sugar, electrolytes, calcium, phosphorus, magnesium.
    - CT scan/MRI of head – depending on the recent medical history of the child.
    - EEG – usually not done emergently.
    - Spinal tap (lumbar puncture) – only if there is a strong suspicion of meningitis.
    - Medications are not normally prescribed for a first (or even second) seizure – but again, treatment options vary depending on the entire clinical picture.
    - Referral of the child is often made to a Pediatric Neurologist for further care (medication decisions, further testing, long term management).

# HEAD LICE:

> A common and not serious problem among school-aged children and then, subsequently, their families. It is not a health hazard and does not suggest uncleanliness or poor hygiene.
> It is a major nuisance for parents.

## CAUSES:

- A parasite that has several stages of life; first, that of a "nit", or egg, followed by a young hatched nymph (young bug), and then finally an adult "bug".

## SYMPTOMS:

- Significant itching of the scalp.

## WHAT TO LOOK FOR:

- Very small pale white to clear "eggs" (nits) located on the hairshafts about one inch above the scalp. They can best be found on the back of the scalp just above the hairline. However, on close inspection, the nits can be found just about anywhere on the scalp. "Live bugs" which are dark in color may be seen crawling around in the hair as well.

### WHEN TO CONTACT YOUR CHILD'S HEALTHCARE PROVIDER

- **When you find nits or live bugs in your child's hair. Your child's healthcare provider can prescribe the medication that is used to treat head lice.**

## WHAT TO DO AT HOME:

- Treatment is usually a lotion that is applied to the hair and left on for a prescribed length of time. It is important to follow the directions that come with the medication. Do not apply any more often than what is directed; these medications can have side effects if not used properly.
- Use a nit comb (which usually comes with the medication) to comb out nits and lice.
- After treatment, check the scalp every 2-3 days for additional nits or live bugs. Remove them if seen.
- Retreatment is recommended 7 days following the initial treatment.
- Continue to check for nits and live bugs for 2 – 3 weeks after treatment is completed.

## IMPORTANT:

- For prevention, encourage your child to not share combs or brushes with others; in addition, do not share hats and scarfs.
- In addition to treating your child, it is also important to decontaminate any clothing, hats, scarfs, towels and bed clothing that the child has come in contact with in the 48 hours prior to treatment. This means washing all bed clothing and clothes in hot water and then drying on high heat cycle. For items that cannot be washed, sealing them in a plastic bag for 2 weeks is recommended.
- The Academy of Pediatrics (AAP) feels that a child with head lice should NOT be restricted from school while waiting for clearance of all nits and live bugs after treatment.
- Source: CDC guidelines, American Academy of Pediatrics.

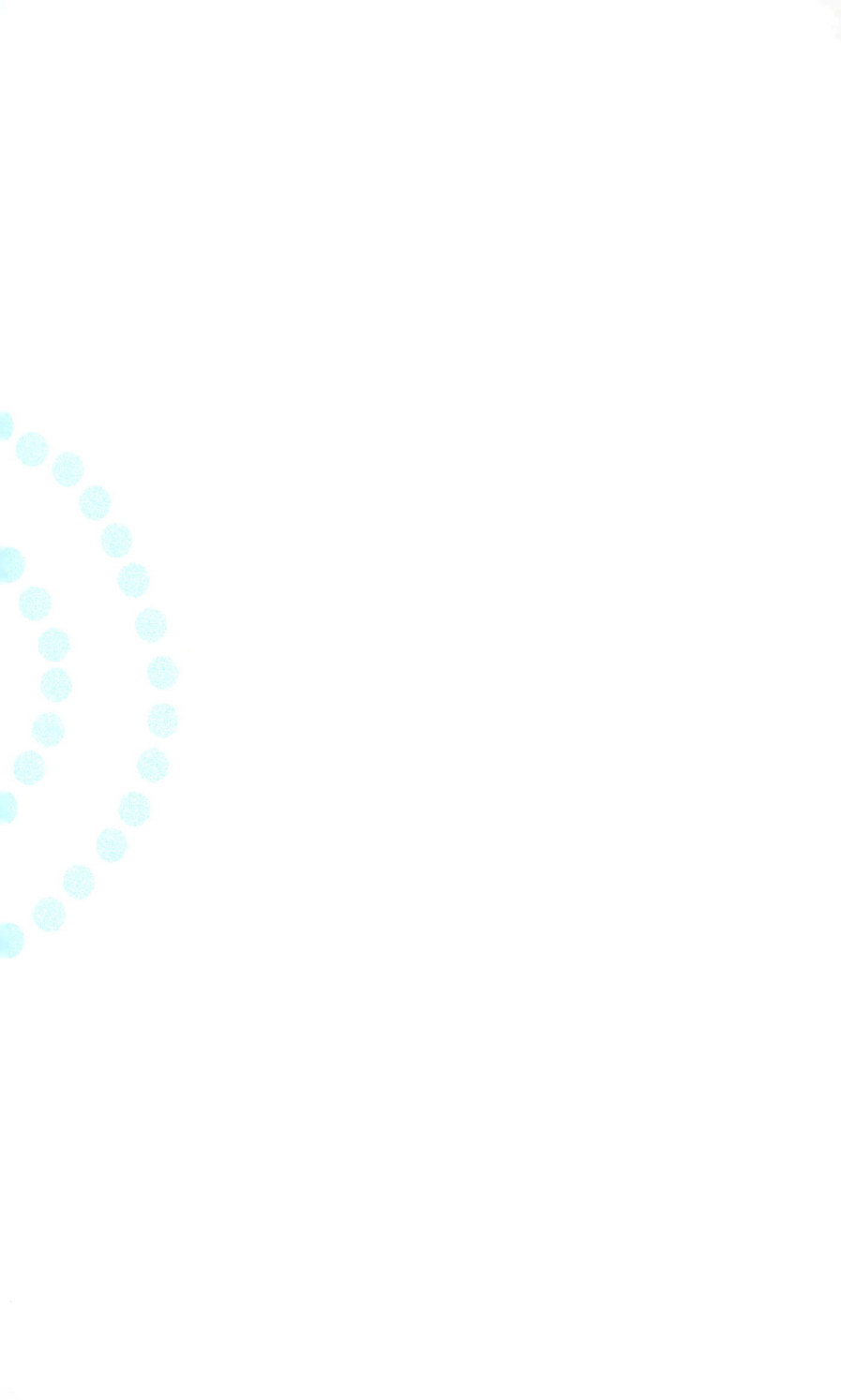

# THE EAR
## CHAPTER 23

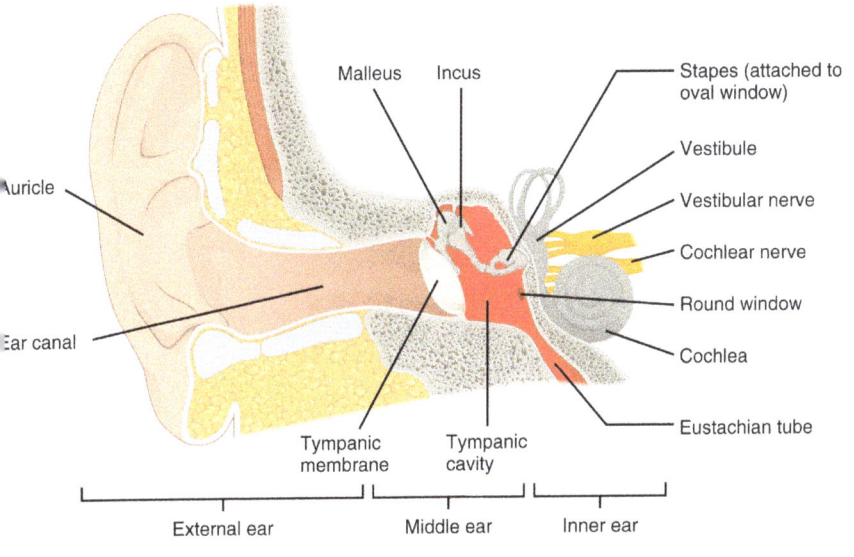

Malleus — Incus — Stapes (attached to oval window) — Vestibule — Vestibular nerve — Cochlear nerve — Round window — Cochlea — Eustachian tube — Tympanic cavity — Tympanic membrane — Ear canal — Auricle — External ear — Middle ear — Inner ear

OpenStax, CC BY 4.0 via Wikimedia Commons

# EAR PAIN:

> Ear pain in children is not uncommon – but not all ear pain is an ear infection.

## CAUSES:

- Ear infections (middle ear infections).
- Swimmer's ear.
- Teething.
- TMJ (temporomandibular joint pain).

## TO BETTER UNDERSTAND EAR PROBLEMS, SOME INTRODUCTION TO THE EAR:

- The middle ear lining routinely produces clear fluid that normally drains "out" through the Eustachian tube into the back of the nose. When a person's eustachian tube becomes blocked (occurs typically when the lining of the eustachian tube becomes swollen during colds or nasal allergies) the fluid builds up in the middle ear space. An additional method of blockage of the eustachian tube is enlarged adenoids covering the tube's opening.
- When there is fluid in the middle ear space, a child's hearing is decreased to a certain extent; the fluid in the middle ear dampens the vibrations of the three bones in the middle ear chamber that transmit vibrations from the ear drum to the inner ear. Once all fluid is gone from the middle ear space, hearing returns to normal.
- The middle ear fluid will drain again on its own once the Eustachian tube opens up – but this can sometimes take several weeks to months.
- Following are common problems associated with ear pain.

# MIDDLE EAR INFECTION (Acute Otitis Media):

More common in infants and toddlers, but can occur in any age.

## Otitis media

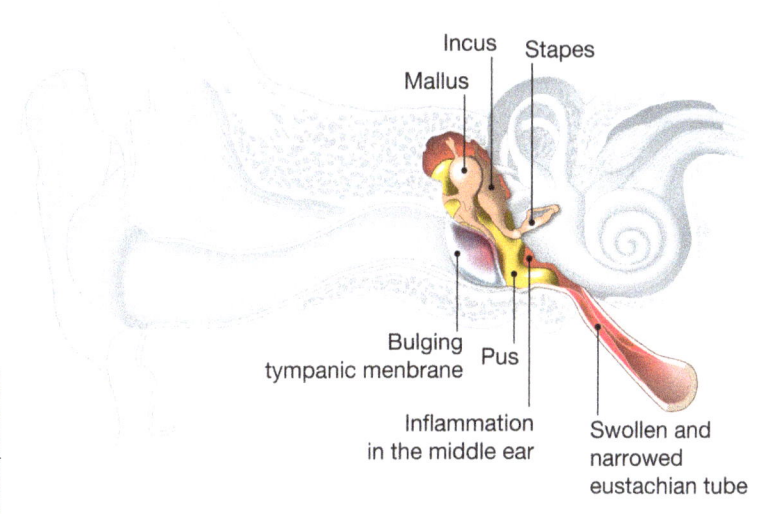

- Incus
- Stapes
- Mallus
- Bulging tympanic menbrane
- Pus
- Inflammation in the middle ear
- Swollen and narrowed eustachian tube

## CAUSES:

- Occurs when accumulated middle ear fluid behind the ear drum becomes infected.
- Bacteria and viruses can both cause ear infections; they get to the middle ear by making their way from the nasal passages through the Eustachian tube and into the middle ear space.
- When there is fluid in the middle ear space, the organisms can create an infection, causing the fluid to become cloudy and thicker.
- The increased pressure in the middle ear as well as the infection itself cause the ear pain.

## SYMPTOMS:

- Pulling at ears (other conditions can cause this as well).
- Crying, irritability.
- Fever.
- Complaints of ear pain.

## WHAT TO DO AT HOME

- Give acetaminophen or ibuprofen for pain (see appendix for dosages).
- Instill ear pain drops into affected ear. (Do not use if your child has ear tubes or ear drainage). Ear pain drops are available at major pharmacy retail departments.
- Make an appointment with your child's medical provider.

### WHEN TO CONTACT YOUR CHILD'S HEALTHCARE PROVIDER

- **When your child complains of ear pain.**
- **Since ear infections are common in infants and toddlers, it is a good idea to be seen at your provider's office where your child's medical records are kept. It is important to track ear infections; if they become recurrent, a decision when to refer to an ear specialist is based upon the frequency of ear infections and the persistence of fluid in the middle ear – all information that will be contained in your child's medical record. (Records from Urgent Care/E.R. are not always shared with your child's provider).**

## DIAGNOSIS AND TREATMENT:

- Made by examination of the ear by qualified medical professionals.
- Antibiotics (oral) are usually prescribed.
- "Watchful waiting" (not prescribing an antibiotic) is done in some situations.

## IMPORTANT:

- Occasionally the ear drum can develop a perforation (or tear) due to marked increased pressure in the middle ear from an ear infection. If this occurs, there will be drainage seen coming from the auditory canal opening. It may be cloudy, clear, colored, or bloody. The perforation is not a serious problem – it actually helps with immediate pain relief because the pressure can be released and the perforation then heals promptly on its own. Antibiotic drops are not indicated if this occurs; the oral antibiotic will be sufficient.

- Referrals are made to an ENT specialist (otolaryngologist) based upon the following:

  - Recurrent ear infections: 3 or more ear infections in 6 months OR 4 infections in one year.

  - Evidence of hearing loss when fluid remains in the middle ear after an infection has been treated.

  - Persistence of fluid behind the ear drum for more than 3 months.

    Guidelines published, February, 2022 American Academy of Otolaryngology.

  - The ENT specialist may recommend placement of ear tubes (tympanostomy tubes) if fluid persists for more than 3 months in infants and toddlers and/or prolonged persistence with hearing loss in older children.
    The recommendation will be based on the history of your child's ear problems and a thorough exam of your child's ears and other surrounding structures.

# OTITIS MEDIA WITH EFFUSION:

> Occurs when the middle ear has accumulated fluid behind the ear drum that is not infected.

## CAUSES:
- Colds (upper respiratory infections).
- Allergies.
- Enlarged adenoids.

## SYMPTOMS:
- A feeling of "pressure" or fullness in the ear.
- A need for the ear to "pop".
- Muffled hearing.
- Infants and toddlers may show no symptoms.

## WHAT TO DO AT HOME:
- Give acetaminophen or ibuprofen for pain (see appendix for dosages).

### WHEN TO CONTACT YOUR CHILD'S HEALTHCARE PROVIDER
- **When your child complains of ear pain.**
- **When you have concerns that your child is not hearing well.**

## DIAGNOSIS AND TREATMENT:

- Is made by examination of the ear by qualified medical professionals.
- Antihistamines/decongestants – theoretically these should help if there are allergy symptoms or an upper respiratory illness (cold), but there is not strong evidence that they really help.
- Steroid nasal sprays (Flonase®, Nasocort®, Nasonex®, Rhinocort®) have been shown to be of benefit in eliminating the fluid more efficiently.
- Time is helpful as well (an acute episode normally resolves in 3 weeks – 3 months).

Children who have nasal symptoms (nasal congestion, runny nose) are more at risk for developing ear infections or middle ear fluid. Minimizing the development of nasal symptoms can decrease the number of ear infections or chronic ear fluid.

How do you do this?

- Insure your home is "smoke-free". Chronic secondhand smoke exposure causes chronic nasal symptoms in children.
- Consider a childcare alternative to a daycare where there are more than 3-4 infants per room. Infants who share their day with more than a few other infants average at least 10 "colds" per year in their first year of attending daycare.

# SWIMMER'S EAR:

Is an infection (usually bacterial) that involves the skin lining the ear canal (auditory canal) that runs from the ear lobe to the ear drum (tympanic membrane)

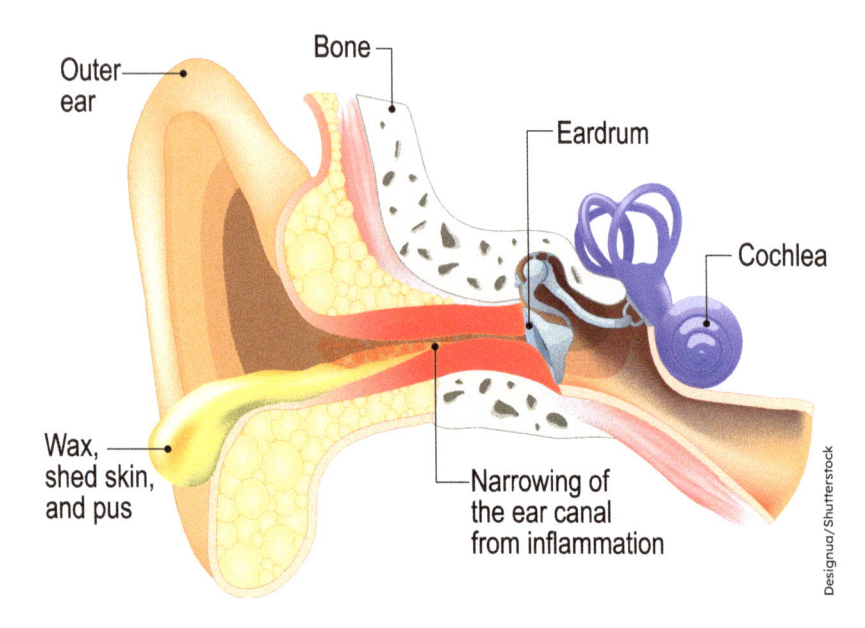

## CAUSES:

- Frequent swimming or any activity that allows significant water into the ear canal, such as swimming in public pools, the ocean, and lakes, can cause "swimmer's ear"(showering and shampooing hair are not considerations here). Another activity that can cause this type of ear infection, especially in younger children, is lying down in bathtub water. Swimming in a private swimming pool is an infrequent cause of "swimmer's ear".

- Prolonged exposure to contaminated water softens the skin lining the auditory canal and makes it easier for bacteria in the water to enter the skin and set up infection.

## SYMPTOMS:

- Ear pain (sometimes worse than middle ear infection pain).
- Pain with tugging on the ear lobe.
- Normally no fever.

## WHAT TO DO AT HOME:

- Treat pain with acetaminophen or ibuprofen (see Appendix for dosages).
- Ear pain drops may be used until the child receives treatment from the healthcare provider. (DO NOT USE if your child has ear tubes)

## DIAGNOSIS AND TREATMENT:

- Direct visualization of the ear canal by a healthcare professional is confirmatory.
- Sometimes the diagnosis is assumed if there is pain with pulling on the ear and a history of recent or frequent swimming.
- Prescription antibiotic ear drops are given for 7 days.
- Pain control with acetaminophen or ibuprofen is usually required until the antibiotic treatment starts to help — which may be 24-48 hours.

## IMPORTANT:

- Prevention is easy.
- Make up a solution of equal parts white vinegar and rubbing alcohol.
- Using a dropper, put 5 drops in each ear after your child is done swimming for the day.
- **DO NOT DO THIS IF YOUR CHILD HAS EAR TUBES!**
- ENT doctors do not recommend ear plugs to prevent Swimmer's Ear infections.

## WHEN TO CONTACT YOUR CHILD'S HEALTHCARE PROVIDER

- **When you suspect this kind of ear infection.**
- **The provider may want to see your child or given the history may just prescribe medication.**

# ADDITIONAL CAUSES OF EAR PAIN:

- **TEETHING:**
  Infants tend to pull on their ears at times during teething. Unfortunately it is impossible to know if there is an ear infection during these times; therefore it would be beneficial to have your child's healthcare provider evaluate your child's ears.

- **TEMPOROMANDIBULAR JOINT PAIN (TMJ):**
  This normally occurs in children older than 10 years of age. The temporamandibular joint sits in very close proximity to the middle ear. It is extremely difficult to decipher where the pain is coming from in this situation.
  The pain in the joint can be caused by changes in teeth orientation over time, excessive chewing of gum, and teeth grinding at night. The pain is helped by ibuprofen as needed; in addition, the dentist may offer a bite guard for nighttime wearing.

- **THROAT PAIN:**
  A sore throat may also cause ear pain at times, thus it is important for your child to have a thorough examination.

# THE EYE
## CHAPTER 3

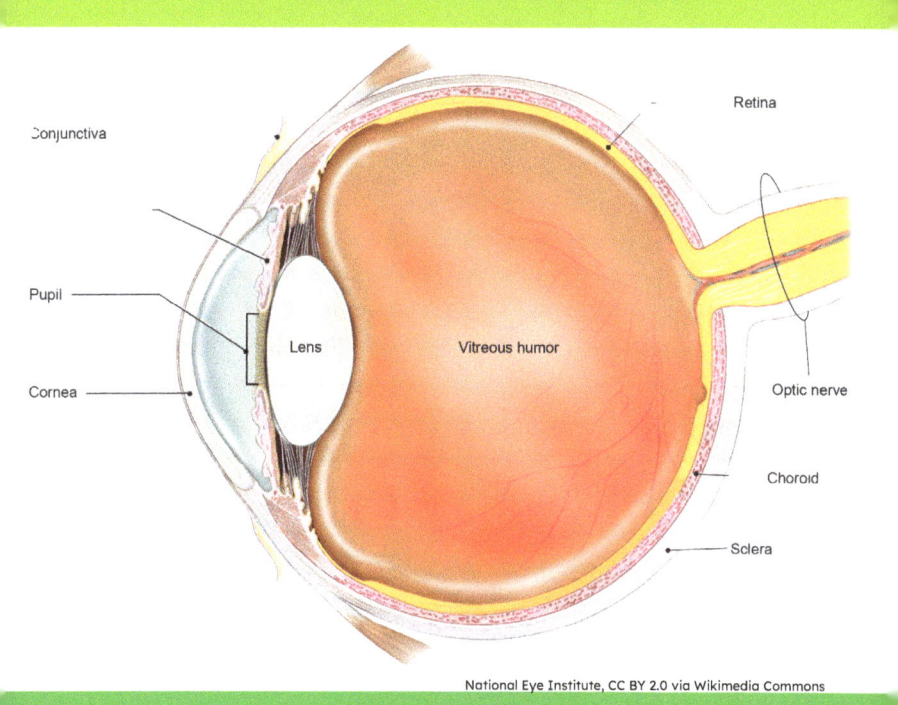

[33]

- Conjunctiva
- Pupil
- Cornea
- Lens
- Vitreous humor
- Retina
- Optic nerve
- Choroid
- Sclera

National Eye Institute, CC BY 2.0 via Wikimedia Commons

# 34 The Eye

# CONJUNCTIVITIS:

> An inflammation, irritation, or infection of the outer surface of the eyeball and the inner surface of the eyelid.

Healthy eye

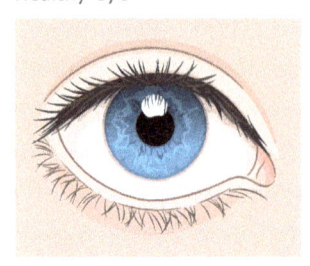

Bacterial conjunctivitis

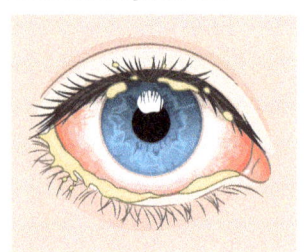

Viral conjunctivitis

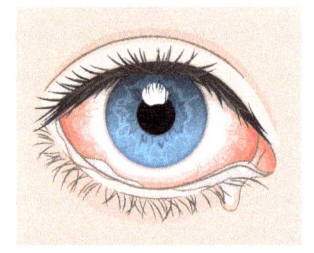

Allergic conjunctivitis

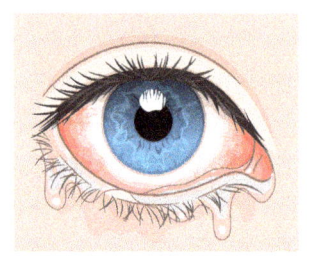

Refluo/Shutterstock

## CAUSES:

- **VIRAL:** white of the eye is pink, watery discharge, goop upon waking up, gritty feeling, eye can itch, often associated with a cold.
- **BACTERIAL:** white of the eye is pink, yellow/green discharge, goop upon awakening and throughout the day, gritty feeling, eye can itch, often associated with a cold.
- **ALLERGIES:** white of the eye is pink, watery discharge, goop upon waking up, gritty feeling, eye can itch, eyelids may be puffy. Occurs during allergies.
- **CHEMICAL:** white of the eye is pink, may have watery discharge, goop upon waking up. Eye can itch or burn. Known exposure, for example, heavily chlorinated pool water.

## WHAT TO DO AT HOME:

- It would be best to contact your child's medical provider to obtain recommendations. The provider will obtain a history and perform a physical examination to make the diagnosis and treatment plan.

## DIAGNOSIS AND TREATMENT:

- **VIRAL:** No antibiotic eye drop required or indicated. Cool, moist compresses held up against the eyes as needed. Can use artificial tear eye drops as needed.
- **BACTERIAL:** antibiotic eye drops or ointment prescribed by a provider. Cool moist compresses held up against the eye as needed.
- **ALLERGIES:** allergy eye drops (available over the counter). Consider giving oral antihistamines as well. Cool, moist compresses held against the eyes as needed. Avoid cause of allergy symptoms (stay inside on bad pollen days).
- **CHEMICAL:** artificial tears. Cool, moist compresses held up against the eyes. Ibuprofen for pain and discomfort.

## IMPORTANT:

- Viral and bacterial conjunctivitis usually improve after 3-5 days, even without antibiotic eye drops.
- Antibiotic eye drops can improve symptoms a bit faster and prevent spread IF it is a bacterial infection.
- Both viral and bacterial eye infections are quite contagious and easily spread among children and family members.
- TO PREVENT SPREADING AN EYE INFECTION – wash hands frequently, keep hands away from eyes (do not rub eyes), do not share wash clothes that have been near eyes.

## 36 The Eye

# CHALAZION:

> A blocked gland that produces tears located in the main part of the eyelid. A bump or lump appears in the eyelid proper. There is associated redness and tenderness to the area. It is not contagious.

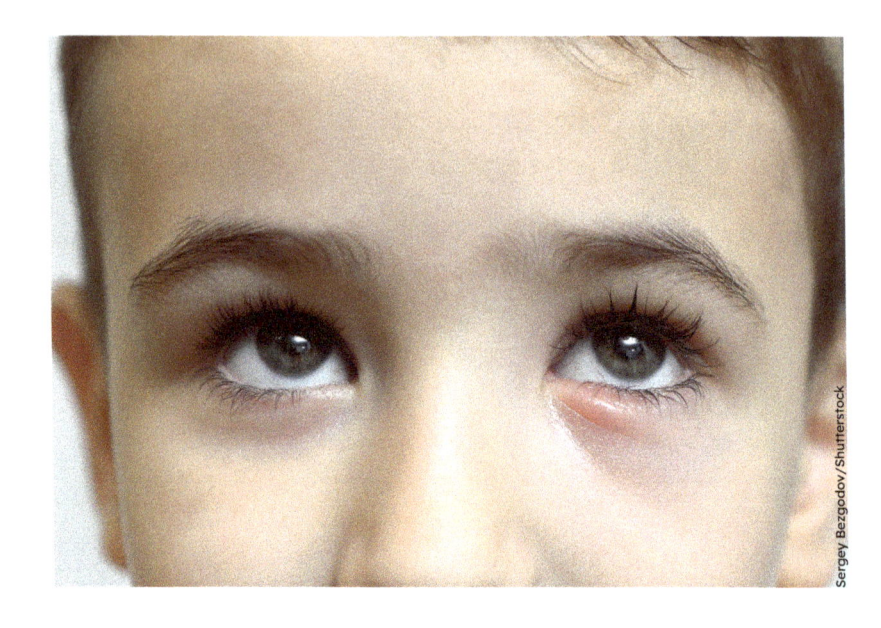

## TREATMENT:

- Warm, moist compresses held up against the area involved.
- If the lump persists for several days, despite the warm compresses, an antibiotic eye ointment or eye drop can be prescribed.
- If the lump persists for several weeks, despite treatment, referral to an eye specialist may be done.

**The Eye** 37

# STYE:

> A blocked oil gland or eyelash follicle along the EYELID EDGE that becomes inflamed (red) and tender. It is not contagious.

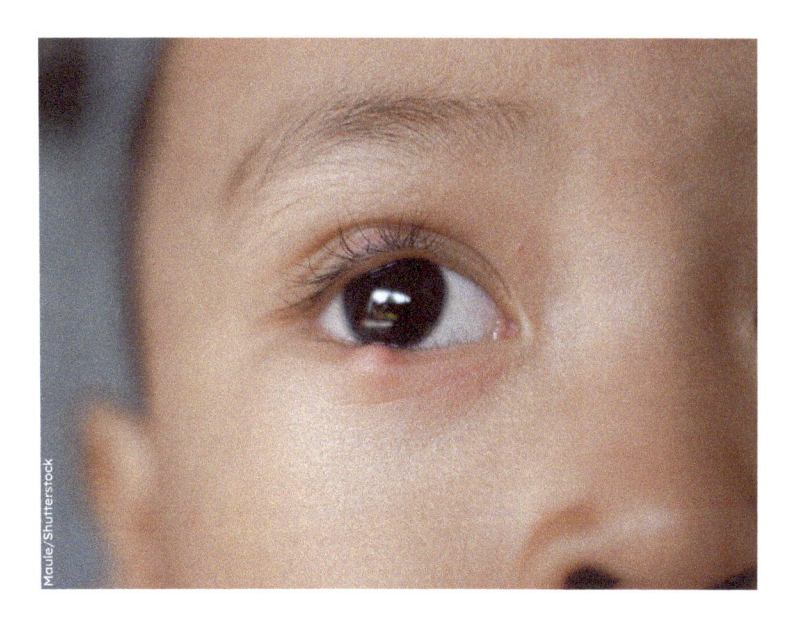

## TREATMENT:

- Warm, moist compresses held up against the stye area for 10-15 minutes, three times a day until gone.
- Antibiotic drops are not necessary.

# EYE SCRATCH:

> These do not happen often, but when they do, they are extremely painful. Consider this as a possibility if your child suddenly starts crying and covers their eye. Ask if anything came close to their eye. Other symptoms include excessive tearing and light sensitivity.

## DIAGNOSIS:

- It can be made by your provider using a special dye put in the corner of the eye and then shining a "black light" in front of the eye that can easily show the scratch.

## TREATMENT:

- Pain control with ibuprofen or acetaminophen.
- Antibiotic eye drops are often prescribed.
- Do not let your child rub the affected eye.
- Eye scratches normally heal on their own over the course of 3-4 days.

## IMPORTANT:

- If the eye does not improve over the next 48-72 hours after the injury (and being seen), re-contact your provider.

### FOR ALL EYE ISSUES: CALL YOUR CHILD'S HEALTHCARE PROVIDER URGENTLY

- **When there is pain in the eye that is new or worsening.**
- **When vision is blurred.**
- **When there is significant light sensitivity.**
- **When there is worsening redness despite using antibiotic eye drops or ointment.**

# THE NOSE

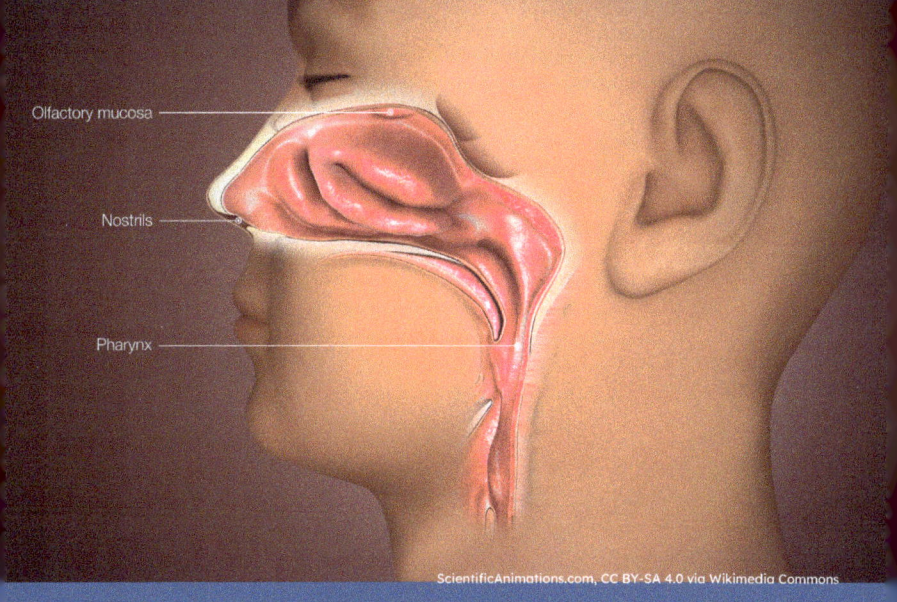

CHAPTER 4

- Olfactory mucosa
- Nostrils
- Pharynx

ScientificAnimations.com, CC BY-SA 4.0 via Wikimedia Commons

# NOSEBLEEDS (EPISTAXIS):

## CAUSES:
- Dry air: it dries out the lining of the nose.
- Significant sneezing/allergies.
- Sometimes a cold.
- Picking the nose.
- Very rarely, a bleeding problem.

## WHAT TO DO AT HOME:
- A cold compress to bridge of nose (this helps the blood vessels going to the nose constrict, which then slows down the bleeding).
- Have the child lean forward a little and breath through the mouth.
- Have the child spit out any blood that may get into the throat area.
- DO NOT LAY YOUR CHILD DOWN.
- DO NOT ALLOW YOUR CHILD TO BLOW THE NOSE.
- Try to keep yourself and your child calm. The more agitated one is, the nose will continue to bleed.
- Humidify the bed area in your child's bedroom every night using a cool mist vaporizer.
- Paint the inside of the child's nostrils with petroleum jelly using a cotton swab; do this 1-2 times daily. This helps to soften and hydrate the lining of the nose so it will not crack and then bleed. Insert the cotton swab in as far as the cotton on the tip.

NOTE: It is common to see passage of clots during a nosebleed; this is not anything to worry about.

## WHEN TO CONTACT YOUR CHILD'S HEALTHCARE PROVIDER

▸ **When your child is having nosebleeds several times a week despite your home therapy.**

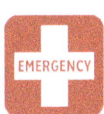

## WHEN TO GO TO THE EMERGENCY ROOM

▸ **When the nosebleed lasts longer than 20-30 minutes, take your child to the Emergency Room for further care.**

---

What exactly causes the nose to bleed? A blood vessel just under the surface of the nasal lining can "pop open" from a variety of reasons.

Bleeding from the nose is not unusual in children and is usually not a sign of anything serious.

Nosebleeds can be associated with high blood pressure – but only in adults.

# UPPER RESPIRATORY ILLNESSES/INFECTIONS: "COLDS"

> Caused by viruses (many different ones), a cold is easily "passed on" to other people (children and adults), and normally occurs in the cooler months of the year. During the first year of attending day care, a child averages 10 different respiratory infections. A cold normally lasts 10-14 days and there is nothing to alter the course. Upper respiratory infections can be associated with ear infections.

## SYMPTOMS:

- Nasal drainage — usually clear, but can be cloudy, yellow or green at times.
- Occasional sneezing.
- A cough caused by postnasal drainage. Mucus drains down the back of the nose, irritates the already irritated lining of the upper respiratory tract from the cold and stimulates the cough receptors, setting off the cough. Coughs from colds and allergies can be worse when lying down due to the fact that mucus drains more/better when we are in that position.
- Fever, but not always.

## WHAT TO DO AT HOME:

- There are NO "cold" medications recommended for children under 6 years of age.
- It is important to suction the nose (in infants) as often as necessary. A bulb syringe (usually sent home from the hospital after your child is born) is very helpful. In addition, you can purchase nasal aspirators that are helpful.
- Prior to suctioning an infant's nose, it is helpful to use some normal saline drops to help loosen mucous and make it easier to suction out. A recipe for normal saline drops can be found in the appendix. Warning: your baby will hate this.
- For older children, make them/help them blow their nose as needed.
- Acetaminophen or ibuprofen can be used to treat any fever associated with a cold or for symptomatic relief.

### WHEN TO CONTACT YOUR CHILD'S HEALTHCARE PROVIDER

- **If you child is not showing improvement after 4-5 days of illness.**
- **If your child has a fever that does not go away after 48-72 hours.**

## PREVENTION:

- Good and frequent hand washing can help reduce trasmission of colds. Keep hands out of eyes.

## IMPORTANT:

- There are really no significant benefits from "cold" or "cough" medications purchased over the counter.
- They are not very helpful in reducing the symptoms of a cold, nor do they cure a cold.
- Children under 6 years of age should not be given any cold or cough medication.

# ALLERGIC RHINITIS (HAY FEVER)

> Can occur with allergic conjunctivitis (eye allergies).
> Can be associated with a cough.
> Can be associated with asthma.
> It is not contagious.
> Normally does not occur in children under one year of age.

## CAUSES:

- Allergens either inside or outside the home.
- Seasonal allergic rhinitis is triggered by outdoor allergens, typically during the spring and fall seasons.
- Inside allergens (dust mites, animal dander, mold) can cause symptoms all year long.

## SYMPTOMS:

- Nasal stuffiness and clear nasal discharge.
- Sneezing.
- Occasional cough.
- The cough is caused by mucus produced in the nasal passages, similar to coughs in Upper Respiratory illnesses.
- No fever.

## IMPORTANT POINTS:

- Keep your child inside on days when his/her specific allergy's pollen count(s) are high.
- Giving an antihistamine on a daily basis is very helpful for preventing or minimizing allergy symptoms, as well as treating acute allergy symptoms.

## The Nose 45

### WHEN TO CONTACT YOUR CHILD'S HEALTHCARE PROVIDER

- **If you have been using one of the medications listed in the next paragraph and your child's symptoms are not improving. Please note that there are additional medications that your child's medical provider may prescribe.**
- **EMERGENCY ROOM VISITS ARE NOT INDICATED FOR ALLERGIC RHINITIS**

## TREATMENT AND DIAGNOSIS:

- Oral antihistamines are the main treatment. There are several options:

  - Benadryl® (diphenhydramine) – is short acting, needs to be given every 4-6 hours; indicated for infants ages 6 months and older.
  - Claritin® (loratadine) – is long acting (once daily), safe for children aged one year and older.
  - Zyrtec® (cetirizine) – is long acting (once daily), safe for children aged one year and older.
  - Allegra® (fexofenadine) - is long acting; indicated for children 2 years and older.

- Nasal steroid sprays:

  - Some examples are: Flonase®, Nasacort®, Nasonex® and Rhinocort®.
  These nasal sprays do not work immediately – they have to be used for several days in a row before they become effective. They are used to control and minimize allergy symptoms.
  Can be purchased over the counter.
  Can safely be used in children two years of age and up. Consult with your provider before starting one of these for your child.

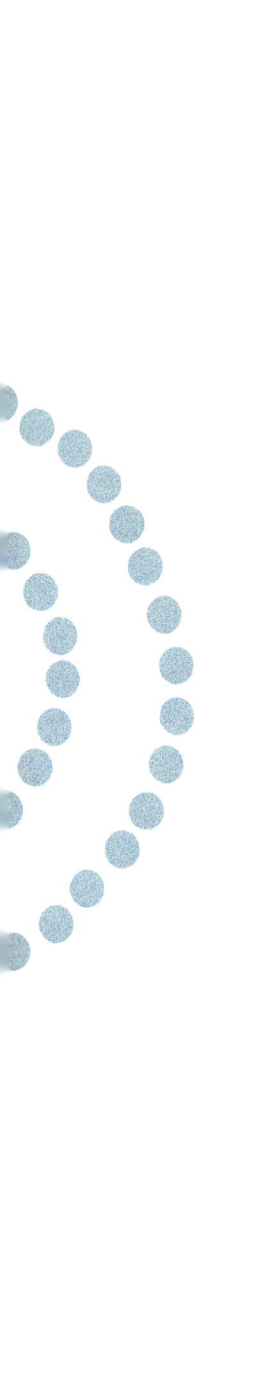

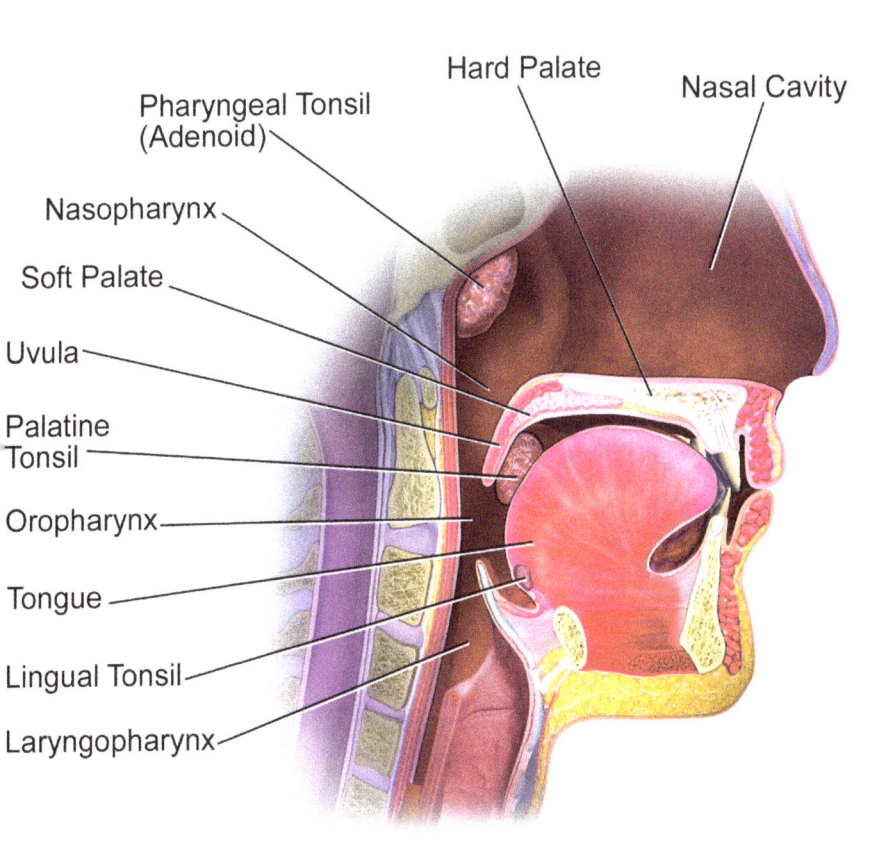

# THE THROAT

**CHAPTER 5**

- Hard Palate
- Nasal Cavity
- Pharyngeal Tonsil (Adenoid)
- Nasopharynx
- Soft Palate
- Uvula
- Palatine Tonsil
- Oropharynx
- Tongue
- Lingual Tonsil
- Laryngopharynx

Blausen.com staff (2014) Medical gallery of Blausen Medical via Wikimedia Commons

# SORE THROAT:

## CAUSES:

- INFECTIONS

    Caused by viruses (the most common cause of sore throats in all age groups) OR bacteria (in particular: Strep bacteria).

- ALLERGY PROBLEMS

    Sore throat will occur during the time of year that one is having allergy issues such as sneezing, runny nose, or stuffy nose. The throat can actually itch in this condition as well.

- DRY THROAT

    This can occur from not drinking enough liquids over the course of the day OR being dehydrated OR sleeping with one's mouth open.

- ACID REFLUX

    Acid made in the stomach to help with digestion can be refluxed up to the throat area.
    This will cause irritation and soreness in the throat.

# The Throat

## NON-SPECIFIC VIRAL INFECTIONS:

> Most common infectious cause of sore throats in all age groups.
> Many non-specific viruses cause sore throats.

## SYMPTOMS:

- Sore throat.
- Nasal symptoms.
- Cough.
- Maybe fever.
- Headache.
- Body aches.

## WHAT TO DO AT HOME:

- Give your child acetaminophen or ibuprofen to help with the throat pain.
- Encourage increase in fluid intake when a sore throat is present.

A specific viral infection: INFLUENZA.

A specific viral respiratory illness whose symptoms include: nasal congestion and discharge, cough, sore throat, body aches and fever (which can be high); the acute phase – including fever - may last 5-10 days.

It is diagnosed by a nasal swab test performed by a medical provider.

Treatment includes: fever control and other comfort measures. Children with chronic medical conditions are candidates for an antiviral medication.

Prevention: the "flu vaccine" can at least minimize or else prevent influenza.

# MONONUCLEOSIS:

> A very specific VIRAL infection caused by the Epstein Barr Virus (EBV).

## SYMPTOMS:

- Sore throat (can be very sore).
- Significant swelling of the lymph nodes in the neck area - front, sides and back.
- Swollen red tonsils with typically a white coating.
- Fever may or may not be present.
- Occasional rash on the trunk and extremities.
- Tiredness out of the ordinary.
- Voice sounds like "speaking with a hot potato in the mouth".

## WHEN TO CONTACT YOUR CHILD'S HEALTHCARE PROVIDER

- **When any of the above symptoms are present.**

## DIAGNOSIS AND TREATMENT:

- Diagnosis is made with a blood test.
- If fever is present, manage it with acetaminophen or ibuprofen.
- Rest — a child may require much more rest/sleep compared to his/her normal amount to recover.
- Increased fluid intake needs to be strongly encouraged.
- Soft foods until throat pain is gone are important.
- IN SOME SITUATIONS, the provider may order oral steroids if the swelling of the tonsils is significant and swallowing is difficult.

# BACTERIAL INFECTIONS - STREP THROAT:

> Strep bacteria are the most common cause of bacterial throat infections.

## SYMPTOMS AND FINDINGS:

- Sore throat.
- Fever - sometimes.
- Headache.
- Typically there are no nasal symptoms or cough associated with it.
- Vomiting, occasionally.
- Spotty redness of the roof of the mouth in front of the uvula.
- Redness of the uvula.
- Enlarged tonsils that are usually red (they do not often have a white coating on them – that is more typical of a viral infection).
- Swollen lymph nodes on the front of the neck.
- Strawberry tongue – not seen all the time. Strawberry tongue is a swollen, red tongue with scattered tiny white spots.

## WHAT TO DO AT HOME:

- Treat the symptoms with acetaminophen or ibuprofen until your child can see his medical provider.

## DIAGNOSIS AND TREATMENT:

- A physical exam can be suggestive of strep throat, but diagnosis is confirmed by a rapid strep test or a throat culture done at your child's medical provider's office.
- Acetaminophen or ibuprofen can be given to help with pain until the prescribed antibiotic helps with symptoms.
- Increased fluid intake is important to help with symptom relief.
- Antibiotics are prescribed (it is VERY important to take the entire prescription).

   NOTE: The reason it is important to complete all the antibiotic given to treat strep throat is to prevent the complications of under – treated/not treated strep throat.
   Those complications include inflammation/irritation of the kidneys or rheumatic fever (a serious inflammation of the heart).

## IMPORTANT:

- It has been suggested that one should throw away their toothbrush after being diagnosed with strep throat. Although there is conflicting data on whether this is necessary, dentists recommend replacing a toothbrush every 3-4 months, so it's probably a good idea to do so regardless.
- Strep throat is uncommon in children under 2 years of age.
-10 – 15% of the pediatric population can test positive for strep when they have NO symptoms; this is referred to as the "carrier state".

This does NOT require treatment. Therefore, if for some reason your child is tested for strep even though he/she has no symptoms of sore throat and the test is positive, one should question if an antibiotic is really needed.

# BACTERIAL INFECTIONS - PERITONSILLAR ABSCESS:

> Much less common than strep throat. Infection is in the tissue NEXT to the tonsil (usually just on one side). Usually caused by the strep bacteria.

## SYMPTOMS AND FINDINGS:

- Sore throat.
- Fever - sometimes.
- Patient talks with a "hot potato voice".
- Redness and swelling on one side of the throat.
- The uvula is usually pushed "off to the side" by the swelling.
- Swollen and tender neck lymph nodes on the same side of the swelling.

## WHAT TO DO AT HOME:

- Treat the symptoms with acetaminophen or ibuprofen until your child can see his medical provider.

## DIAGNOSIS AND TREATMENT:

- Strep test is sometimes negative.
- Physical exam is THE MOST important tool to diagnose this condition.
- Often the abscess needs to be drained (usually done in the Emergency Room)
- Antibiotics are always prescribed.

## ALLERGIES:

- Sore throat can occasionally be present when a child is experiencing allergy issues.
- The throat and the roof of the mouth may be very itchy at times as well.
- Other symptoms present could be sneezing, runny/stuffy nose, or cough.
- Fever would be absent.

### DIAGNOSIS AND TREATMENT:

- Use of allergy medications (Allegra®, Claritin®, Zyrtec®).
- Increase the fluid intake during this time.
- Avoidance of what is causing the allergy symptoms.

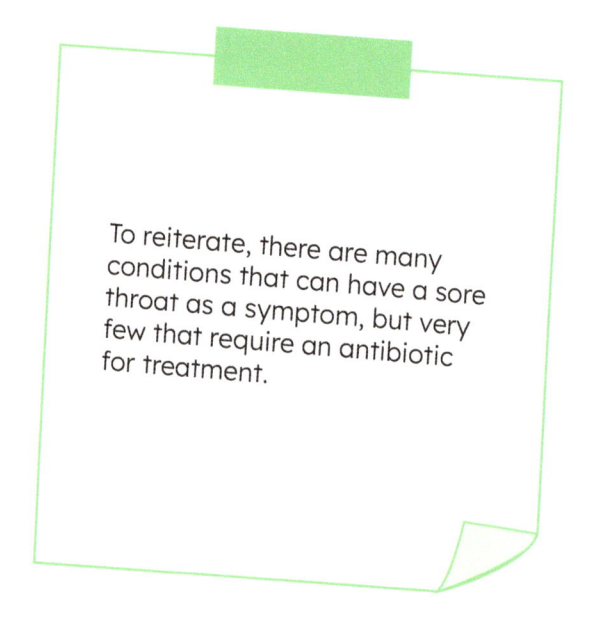

To reiterate, there are many conditions that can have a sore throat as a symptom, but very few that require an antibiotic for treatment.

# ACID REFLUX (GASTRO ESOPHAGEAL REFLUX):

> Usually more common in older children and teenagers. Think about this as a possibility if sore throat complaints last more than a week and the complaints come and go during that time.

## SYMPTOMS:

- Sore throat that may not be present all day, but may come and go throughout the day.

## DIAGNOSIS AND TREATMENT:

- The child's medical provider will take a history and perform a physical exam to aid in making the diagnosis.
- Testing for strep infection is negative.

### TREATMENT:

- Sometimes an acid reducer is recommended by the medical provider.

### LIFESTYLE CHANGES THAT ARE A VERY IMPORTANT PART OF TREATMENT:

- Minimize or do not drink carbonated beverages.
- Minimize or do not drink caffeine beverages.
- Do not eat or drink within 2 hours of going to bed.
- Elevate the head of the bed by 4 inches (this can be done by putting some blocks under the legs at the head of the bed.
- Do not sleep on one's stomach.

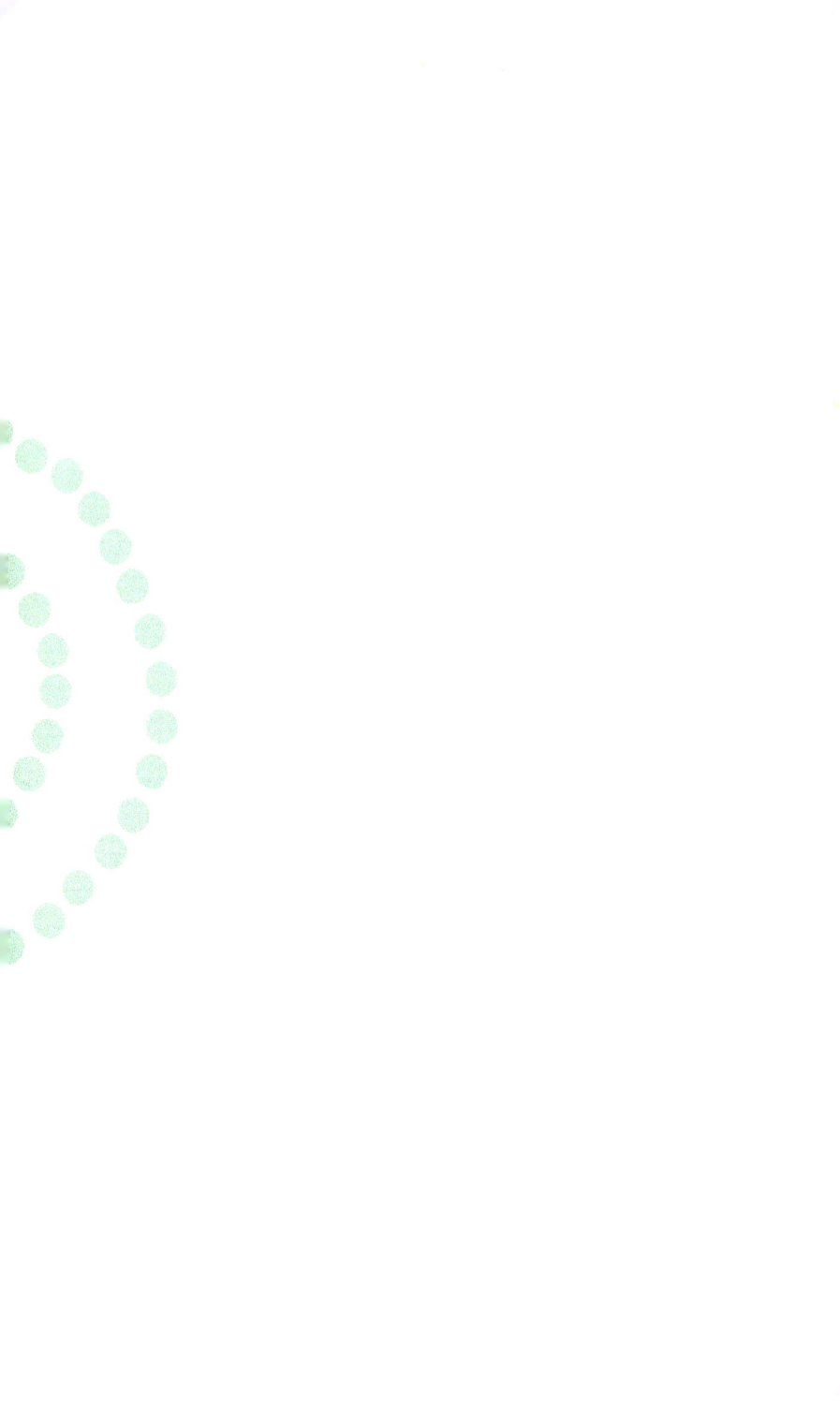

# THE CHEST

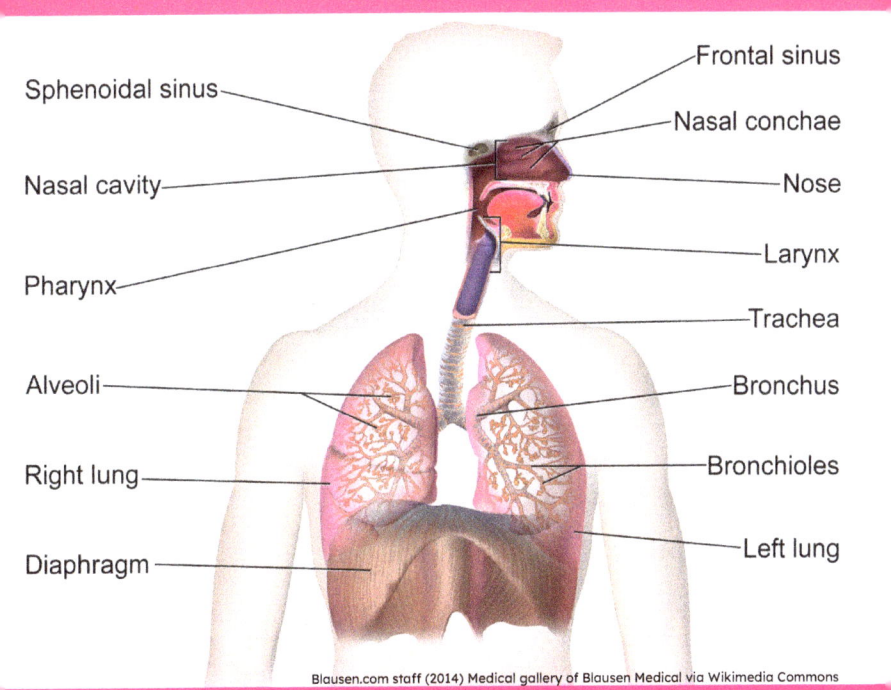

**CHAPTER 6**

57

- Frontal sinus
- Sphenoidal sinus
- Nasal conchae
- Nasal cavity
- Nose
- Pharynx
- Larynx
- Trachea
- Alveoli
- Bronchus
- Right lung
- Bronchioles
- Diaphragm
- Left lung

Blausen.com staff (2014) Medical gallery of Blausen Medical via Wikimedia Commons

# COUGHS AND WHAT CAUSES THEM

> A cough is actually a protective mechanism that the body has to move and clear mucus, as well as other harmful items like food, liquid, stomach acid and other particles from the lower respiratory tract. There is not a single good cough medicine to use in children – in fact, any cough medicine is contraindicated in children under 6 years of age. Coughs from "colds" are going to last 2-3 weeks.

## CAUSES:

- UPPER RESPIRATORY ILLNESSES (COLDS) - See Nose chapter for details.
- CROUP.
- LOWER RESPIRATORY ILLNESSES:
    - Bronchiolitis
    - Pneumonia
    - Asthma
- ALLERGIC RHINITIS (HAY FEVER) - See Nose chapter.
- GASTROESOPHAGEAL REFLUX DISEASE (GERD).

# UPPER RESPIRATORY ILLNESSES (COLDS):

## TREATMENT:

- When the cough is from irritation in the upper respiratory tract (a cold or allergies), honey can help calm the cough momentarily. Honey is safe for any child above one year of age. One teaspoon is a good dose to try. Honey coats the throat and temporarily minimizes the irritation in the area, thus minimizing the cough.
- Cough drops, a steam shower, and gargling with saltwater are all helpful suggestions for older children.

# CROUP

> More common in children under two years of age, but can occur in older children as well.

## CAUSES:

- Viruses that cause croup: parainfluenza, RSV (Respiratory Synctitial Virus), adenovirus, and Covid-19.
- The virus causes inflammation (and thus swelling) of the lower part of the trachea (windpipe), the voice box, and upper bronchial tree of the lungs.

## SYMPTOMS:

- Usually starts in the middle of the night, after the child went to bed fine.
- May have fever.
- Child sometimes acts scared.
- There are 3 distinct sounds that croup causes: barky cough, hoarseness, and stridor (a harsh noise as a child breathes in).
- Cough comes from inflammation caused by the virus.
- The sounds are often more impressive than the degree of seriousness of the condition.
- Can vary in severity amongst children, but hospitalization due to croup is not common.
- The first three days are usually the worst; the condition improves from that time.

## WHAT TO DO AT HOME:

- Look for any respiratory distress:

    - Breathing rate more than 40 times/minute.
    - Nostrils "flaring".
    - "Sucking in" with each breath – in between ribs and under the rib cage.
  
  **\*All of the above need to be looked for while the infant/child is NOT crying or upset\*.**

- Try to keep your child calm (all sounds will improve when child is more relaxed).
- Treat any fever.
- Encourage more fluid intake.
- Steam showers can be helpful in the acute setting of significant coughing "fits".
- Exposure to cool night outdoor air can be helpful as well in an acute setting of significant coughing "fits".

### WHEN TO CONTACT YOUR CHILD'S HEALTHCARE PROVIDER

- **If you see signs of respiratory distress, call your child's medical provider immediately or go to the Emergency Room.**
- **If your child has fever, is acting like he/she is not feeling well, or is not drinking normal amounts, contact your child's medical provider.**

## DIAGNOSIS AND TREATMENT:

- A physical examination by the child's medical provider and hearing the characteristic "bark", hoarseness and stridor confirms the diagnosis.
- Testing is not necessary for diagnosis.
- In some cases of croup, the provider will order oral steroids. This is to help decrease the swelling of the windpipe faster than what it would normally take.
- No antibiotic is indicated.
- Mild cases of croup do not need any treatment.

# Lower Respiratory Illnesses: BRONCHIOLITIS

> More common in children under 2 years of age.
>
> There are now two options available to minimize the severity of RSV infections in infants:
> - An RSV vaccine for expectant mothers during later pregnancy.
> - An injection of RSV antibodies for infants less than 8 months of age.
>
> These are given in timely conjunction with the RSV season.

## CAUSES:

- Viruses that cause bronchiolitis: Respiratory Syncytial Virus (RSV), Human metapneumovirs (HMPV), others.
- Usually occurs in the colder months of the year.
- It is a contagious condition and it is easily transmitted from one child to another.

## SYMPTOMS:

- May have nasal symptoms.
- Cough most prominent symptom – very dry and frequent.
- The cough comes from irritation of the lining of the bronchial system (the breathing tubes in our lungs).
- Wheezing and/or "crackles" can be present.
- Fever may be present.
- The child may have breathing difficulties.
- The severity of the illness can vary from very mild to very serious.
- Normally lasts 10 -14 days.

## WHAT TO DO AT HOME:

- Look for any respiratory distress:

    - Breathing rate more than 40 times/minute
    - Nostrils "flaring"
    - "Sucking in" with each breath – in between ribs and under the rib cage.
  ***All of the above needs to be looked for while the infant/child is NOT crying or upset*.**

## DIAGNOSIS AND TREATMENT:

- Testing for RSV can be done by the provider using a nasal swab.
- Physical exam by the provider usually helps formulate the diagnosis.
- Chest Xrays are not helpful in this situation and are not indicated.
- Treat any fever using acetaminophen or ibuprofen.
- Antibiotics are not indicated.
- Even if the child is wheezing, current guidelines do not recommend routine use of albuterol. It is felt that younger infants do not have the receptors in their lungs to recognize the albuterol, therefore it may not be effective for bronchiolitis.
- The provider may sometimes do a trial treatment of albuterol, but if there is no improvement, it may not be prescribed.
- Steroids are not indicated.
- If the child's oxygen level is low (below 93 %), supplemental oxygen is provided continuously until the level returns to normal.
- If the child needs supplemental oxygen and/or is not taking in adequate fluids to maintain hydration, hospital admission is indicated. Otherwise, the child can be cared for at home.

## The Chest

### WHEN TO CONTACT YOUR CHILD'S HEALTHCARE PROVIDER

- **If you suspect bronchiolitis, it is a good idea to have your child evaluated**
- **If your child is having signs of respiratory distress, call urgently.**
- **If your child has already been evaluated, but you feel that there has been no improvement after 24-48 hours.**

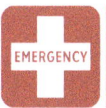

### WHEN TO CALL 911 or GO TO THE EMERGENCY ROOM

- **If there is evidence of respiratory distress in your child and your child's provider is not available, go to the Emergency Room.**

**BRONCHIOLITIS**

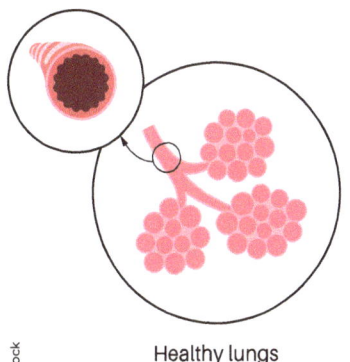

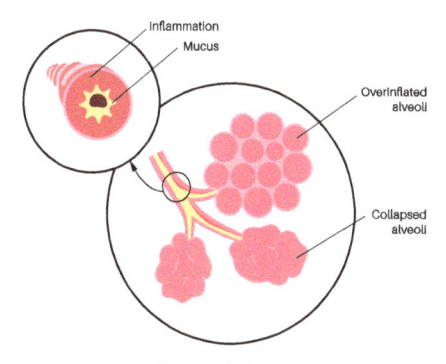

Healthy lungs

Clogged airways

# Lower Respiratory Illnesses: PNEUMONIA

> Fortunately, does not occur often in children.
> Can affect any age group.
> Usually occurs more in the colder months of the year, but can be seen throughout the year.
> Normally it is not a contagious infection.

## CAUSES:

- Main causes are bacteria and viruses.

## SYMPTOMS:

- Cough – either dry "staccato type" or "wet".

- The cough comes from the irritation of the lining of the bronchial system. In this case, the irritation can be caused by a virus or a bacteria.

- Fever may be present.

- Does not necessarily have upper respiratory symptoms (nasal symptoms).

- There may be complaints of chest pain.

- The child may have shortness of breath.

## WHAT TO DO AT HOME:

- Look for any respiratory distress:

    - Breathing rate more than 40 times/minute (in children 5 years and younger) or more than 30 times/minute (in children older than 5 years of age).
    - Nostrils "flaring".
    - "Sucking in" with each breath – in between ribs and under the rib cage.
    
    **\*All of the above need to be looked for while the infant/child is NOT crying or upset\*.**

## WHEN TO CONTACT YOUR CHILD'S HEALTHCARE PROVIDER

- If you suspect pneumonia, it is a good idea to have your child evaluated.
- If your child is having signs of respiratory distress, call urgently.
- If your child has already been evaluated, but you feel that there has been no improvement after 24-48 hours of treatment.

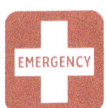

## WHEN TO CALL 911 or GO TO THE EMERGENCY ROOM

- If there is evidence of respiratory distress in your child and your child's provider is not available, go to the Emergency Room.

# DIAGNOSIS AND TREATMENT:

- Can be confirmed by physical exam and sometimes with help of chest Xray.
- Child's oxygen level is usually checked.
- Blood tests are sometimes done to further evaluate the situation.
- Antibiotic is generally prescribed.
- Hospitalization is necessary if the child's oxygen level is low or fluid intake is poor.
- Most cases of pneumonia can be treated at home.
- ** In general, after one has had a pneumonia, a child is NOT more likely to have repeated episodes of pneumonia.**.

# Lower Respiratory Illnesses: ASTHMA (REACTIVE AIRWAY DISEASE)

> A condition involving the airways (breathing tubes) of the lungs - the airways shrink in their overall diameter and the lining of the tubes becomes swollen, thus creating a much smaller space through which air can move.

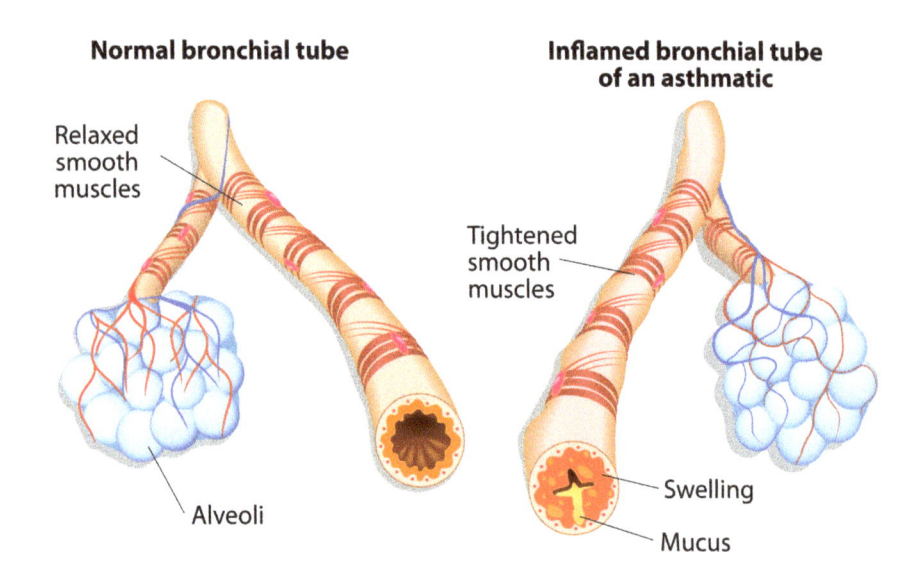

**Normal bronchial tube**
- Relaxed smooth muscles
- Alveoli

**Inflamed bronchial tube of an asthmatic**
- Tightened smooth muscles
- Swelling
- Mucus

Designua/Shutterstock

NOTE: The decrease in size of the airway is what leads to the cough, shortness of breath, and ultimately wheezing that are symptoms (and signs) of asthma.

## CAUSES:

- In younger children (under 5 years of age) the main cause for asthma is a viral respiratory infection.
- In older children (over 5 years of age) the main cause for asthma is most often seasonal and environmental allergies.
- Of course, there are exceptions to the above.

## SYMPTOMS:

- Cough.
- Wheezing
- Shortness of breath.
- Breathing faster.
- Retractions – "sucking in" – in between the ribs while breathing.
- No fever unless there is an associated infection.

## WHAT TO DO AT HOME:

- Look for any respiratory distress:
    - Breathing rate more than 40 times/minute.
    - Nostrils "flaring".
    - "Sucking in" with each breath – in between ribs and under the rib cage.
  
  ***All of the above need to be looked for while the infant/child is NOT crying or upset*.**

## WHEN TO CONTACT YOUR CHILD'S HEALTHCARE PROVIDER

- If this is the first time that you have noticed any of the above symptoms, call your child's medical provider and make an appointment for your child to be evaluated promptly.
- If your child already has a diagnosis of asthma, follow your child's Asthma Action Plan that was provided by your child's provider. If you have any questions regarding the treatment plan, call the medical provider.
- If you hear wheezing, but there is no evidence of respiratory distress.
- If, with wheezing, your child is not eating or drinking very well compared to normal.
- If, with wheezing, your child has a fever that does not improve after 48-72 hours.

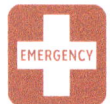

## WHEN TO CALL 911 or GO TO THE EMERGENCY ROOM

- If there is any evidence of respiratory distress and if your provider does not currently have office hours, go to the E.R.

## DIAGNOSIS AND TREATMENT:

- The healthcare provider will take a history and perform a physical exam that will help in the diagnosis of asthma.
- There are no "tests" that can be done in children to diagnose asthma; occasionally, an adult will have a Pulmonary Function Test (PFT) to help in the diagnosis. PFTs are too difficult for most children to accurately complete.
- Asthma is not diagnosed the first time a person wheezes; having recurrent wheezing episodes helps solidify the diagnosis.

## MEDICATIONS FOR ASTHMA:

- Albuterol (by inhaler or nebulizer) - referred to as "Rescue" medication. Albuterol helps the airways expand back to their normal size.
- Steroids orally (for short 5 day courses).
- Steroid (by inhaler or nebulizer) - referred to as "Controller" medication. Steroids help decrease the swelling of the lining of the airways.
- Combination long acting albuterol/steroid inhaler - referred to as " Controller inhaler".
- An "Asthma Action Plan" is a specific asthma management plan put together specifically for your child and should be followed by all who have your child in their care - babysitters, school personnel, camp personnel, coaches, etc.  It is a medication "plan" for your child's overall asthma condition at any one time.

## IMPORTANT:

- Your child's asthma should be regularly managed either by your child's healthcare provider or an asthma specialist. Dosages of medication may need to be increased or decreased depending on how your child overall is doing. Most importantly, please call these providers for recommendations if your child is having asthma flares.

# GASTROESOPHAGEAL REFLUX DISEASE (GERD):

- The cough comes from irritation of the trachea (windpipe) by stomach acid that has been inadvertently inhaled as it moves upward from the stomach. As a person breathes in, acid in the esophagus can be "sucked" into the windpipe. The person immediately coughs when this occurs as a protective mechanism; some acid may not be expelled and will irritate the lining of the windpipe causing a cough.
- In addition, some acid may make it all the way down the vocal cords, irritating them and causing hoarseness.
- Please read the more detailed GASTROESOPHAGEAL REFLUX section in this book in Chapter 8: "The Abdomen".

## SOME FINAL SUGGESTIONS FOR COUGHS IN GENERAL:

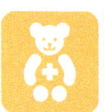

### WHEN TO CONTACT YOUR CHILD'S HEALTHCARE PROVIDER

- **A cough is present for 3 weeks and not improving.**
- **A cough is worsening despite treatment.**
- **There are associated breathing problems associated with the cough.**
- **There is associated fever with the cough.**
- **There is blood being produced by the cough.**

# Other chest issues: BREAST BUDS

> Common in both boys and girls during infancy (usually have disappeared by 6 months but can be present up to 2 years of age) and again after 7-8 years of age.

## CAUSES:
- The cause is hormonal.

## SYMPTOMS:
- A rubbery disc-like object easily felt under the nipple and areola; freely moveable.
- Size of bud does not exceed the size of the areola that it lies under.
- May be tender.
- May just be on one side.

## WHAT TO DO AT HOME:
- Observation only.

### WHEN TO CONTACT YOUR CHILD'S HEALTHCARE PROVIDER

- **If you find one in your child after age 2 years but before age 8 years (this would be a non-emergent visit).**
- **If there is any drainage coming from the nipple.**
- **If the nipple and surrounding skin around the nipple area is very red.**

## DIAGNOSIS AND TREATMENT:

- Your child's provider will do a physical exam; the physical exam can confirm the diagnosis of a breast bud.
- It is rare, but possible, that some girls younger than 8 years of age may start puberty (precocious puberty) earlier than expected (in the range of 4 – 7 years of age) and further laboratory evaluation may be needed. Most of the time, breast buds in girls in this age range are not associated with premature puberty.
- Breast buds are seen in boys anytime after 8 years of age; they can be just on one side or both. They may last up to 6 months before going away. Occasionally, they may not go away.
- Testing or further evaluation of breast buds in boys is rarely needed.

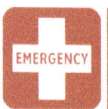

## WHEN TO CALL 911 or GO TO THE EMERGENCY ROOM

- **This condition should not require a 911 call or a visit to the Emergency Room.**

# Other chest issues: CHEST WALL DEFECTS

> A fair number of children can have minor structural differences involving the front part of the chest.

## CAUSES:
- The cause is a person's genetic makeup.

## SYMPTOMS/FINDINGS:
- The sternum (breastbone) may curve outward more than normal (pigeon chest).
- The very lower end of the sternum may "flip up" a little, causing a protrusion or pointed area.
- The very lower end of the sternum may "flip down" a little, causing an indentation.
- The lower third of the sternum may curve inward causing a slightly bigger indentation (pectus excavatum).

## WHAT TO DO AT HOME:
- Observation only.

### WHEN TO CONTACT YOUR CHILD'S HEALTHCARE PROVIDER
- **Your child's routine wellness visit with the provider is an ideal time to assess this condition.**
- **This condition should never require an Emergency Room evaluation.**

## WHAT IS DONE TO EVALUATE/DIAGNOSE/TREAT THIS CONDITION:
- In situations where there is a significant depression of the lower sternum, a referral to a specialist who deals with this condition may be recommended.

# Other chest issues: CHEST PAIN

> Not unusual for a child to complain of chest pain. A heart problem is rarely the cause of chest pain in children and adolescents.

## CAUSES:

- Chest wall pain:

    - the muscles of the chest wall and the rib "joints" (where the ribs connect to the breastbone) are the two components of the chest where pain can originate. Chest wall muscles or the joints can be achy or sore from being over-used in certain situations such as exercise, coughing or vomiting.
    If taking a deep breath reproduces the pain, it is most likely chest wall pain that is the cause of the chest pain.

- Gastroesophageal Reflux Disease:

    - This can cause a pain underneath the breastbone (sternum). The source of the pain is an irritated esophagus caused by stomach acid.
    This is discussed in more detail under Gastroesophageal Reflux Syndrome in the Abdomen section.

- Direct trauma to the chest:

    - Examples: chest injury during a sports activity, a bicycle accident, falling onto an object striking the chest.

## WHAT TO DO AT HOME:

- If you confirm that the source of pain is chest wall pain, a trial of acetaminophen or ibuprofen would be appropriate. Please see appendix for dosages.
- If you confirm that the pain is coming from gastroesophageal reflux disease, a trial of Maalox® or Mylanta® is appropriate. See dosages in appendix. Also see section on GERD.
- Pain from trauma to the chest may respond to ibuprofen or acetaminophen.

## WHEN TO CONTACT YOUR CHILD'S HEALTHCARE PROVIDER

- **When you are concerned and need clarification of the source of the chest pain.**

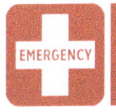

## WHEN TO GO TO THE EMERGENCY ROOM

- **It is usually not necessary to take your child to the Emergency Room for chest pain, unless there is significant pain secondary to an injury of the chest.**

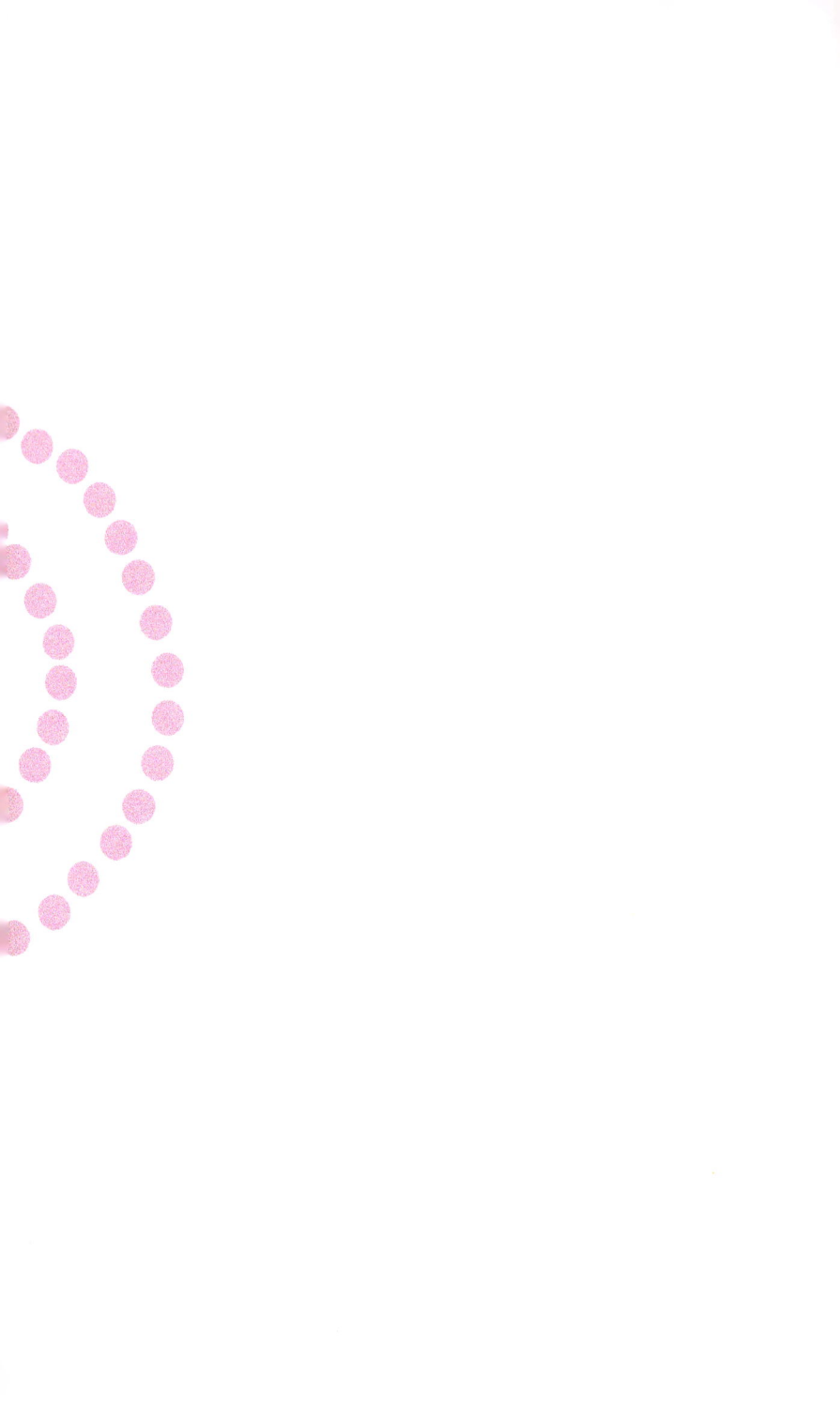

# THE HEART

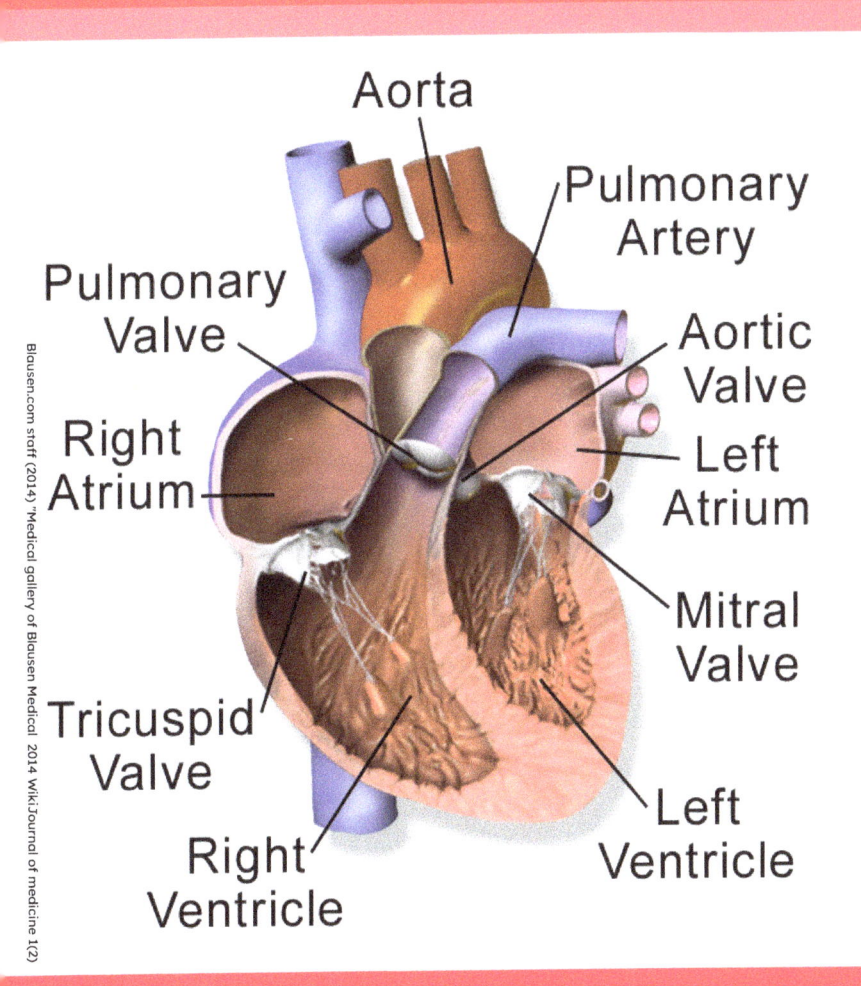

## CHAPTER 7

Aorta

Pulmonary Artery

Pulmonary Valve

Aortic Valve

Right Atrium

Left Atrium

Mitral Valve

Tricuspid Valve

Left Ventricle

Right Ventricle

Blausen.com staff (2014) "Medical gallery of Blausen Medical 2014 WikiJournal of medicine 1(2)

# TACHYCARDIA

> When a child's heart rate is faster than normal.

## CAUSES:

- Fever.
- Increased physical activity.
- Emotional stress/distress.
- Dehydration.
- Some medications.

## SYMPTOMS:

- Your child may not notice anything.
- There may be complaints of the chest pounding.
- Feeling like the heart is going to "jump out of the chest".

## WHAT TO DO AT HOME:

- Count your child's heart rate:

    - To check your child's heart rate, find a good pulse to feel (in children under 2 years, the groin crease has an easy pulse to feel; in children older than 2 years, the pulse in the wrist is easy to find).

    Count the the number of heart beats over 15 seconds and then multiply by 4. This will give you the Beats Per Minute. As the heart rate goes faster, it becomes a little more difficult to count.

    <u>Make sure that your child is in a resting, calm state to get the most accurate heart rate.</u>

## The Heart

## WHAT TO DO AT HOME:

- WHAT HEART RATE IS TOO FAST AND NEEDS TO BE FURTHER EVALUATED?

    - Greater than 160 beats per minute in a child less than one year of age.

    - Greater than 150 beats per minute in a child 12-24 months of age.

    - Greater than 140 beats per minute in a child 2-4 years of age.

    - Greater than 120 beats per minute in a child 4 years and older.

- If your child has a fever, treat it with your choice of acetaminophen or ibuprofen. Recheck the heart rate in 1-2 hours; if the heart rate returns to normal with fever control, continued management of the fever would be the most important action to take.
- If your child has been quite active, encourage rest for awhile and recheck the heart rate. If the rate returns to normal with rest, no further action is needed.
- If your child has been ill with vomiting/diarrhea, encourage more fluid intake.
- If your child is quite anxious, try to resolve what is causing the anxiety. If the anxiety is recurrent, make an appointment to have your child evaluated by the child's provider on a non-emergent basis.

## WHEN TO CONTACT YOUR CHILD'S HEALTHCARE PROVIDER URGENTLY

- If you find that your child's heart rate is faster than the above values, and it has not returned to normal after several hours despite the above recommendations, call your child's medical provider immediately.

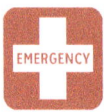

## WHEN TO CALL 911 or GO TO THE EMERGENCY ROOM

- If you find that your child's heart rate is faster than the above values, and you cannot contact your child's provider, go to the Emergency Room.

# DIAGNOSIS AND TREATMENT:

- The provider will take careful history and perform a physical exam.
- Laboratory tests – depending on the situation.
- EKG (ECG/Electrocardiogram)– depending on the situation.
- Treatment will be dependent on the diagnosis.

# SYNCOPE (FAINTING)

> A sudden loss of consciousness as well as loss of motor tone (body becomes limp) caused by the involuntary nervous system – then followed by a rapid and complete recovery.

## CAUSES:

- Caused by a decrease in blood flow to the brain.
- Situations that can lead to this:

    - The site of blood.
    - A very painful experience – ie, smashing your finger.
    - Being dehydrated.
    - Low blood sugar.
    - Standing up too quickly from a lying down or sitting position.
    - Standing for a long time.

## WHAT TO DO AT HOME:

- Place the child flat on the floor or a good supporting surface.
- Lift the legs off the floor (this helps blood from the legs return faster to the heart which then pumps more blood going to the brain).
- Encourage fluid intake after the event
- It is not recommended to give the child a sugary drink or something sweet to eat in this situation; pushing fluids like water or an electrolyte drink would be ideal. A snack consisting of some protein and carbohydrate (i.e. cheese and crackers, pretzels and peanut butter) would be ideal as well, if available.

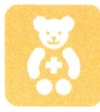

## WHEN TO CONTACT YOUR CHILD'S HEALTHCARE PROVIDER

- Most episodes of fainting are not due to a serious problem, but it is important – at least with the first episode – to have your child seen and evaluated.
- If the episode of fainting would occur during physical activity, it IS very important to have your child evaluated immediately. Fainting during physical activity suggests a possible cardiac abnormality.

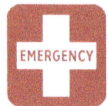

## WHEN TO CALL 911 or GO TO THE EMERGENCY ROOM

- **If the episode of fainting occurs during physical activity, your child should be evaluated in the Emergency Room URGENTLY.**

## WHAT WILL BE DONE TO EVALUATE/TREAT THE PROBLEM:

- The provider will obtain further history and perform a physical exam.
    - Laboratory tests may be performed.
    - An EKG may be performed.
    - A referral to a pediatric cardiologist may be suggested.

## PREVENTION:

- Ensure that your child always drinks adequate amounts of fluids daily; water and milk are the most important fluids for one to drink.
- Make sure that your child's school will allow your child to drink liquids (water) throughout the day
- If your child has fainted before when getting up too quickly, teach the child how to get up in a more controlled manner.
- If your child has fainted before while standing for awhile, teach the child how to shift weight back and forth between the feet and tightening the leg muscles. These are all methods to keep the blood flowing in and out of the leg blood vessels, and preventing blood from pooling in the legs.
- Instruct your child to sit down or lay down as soon as possible if starting to feel faint.

## IMPORTANT POINTS:

- Fainting seldom occurs before 8 years of age.
- Very seldom is there a problem with the heart.

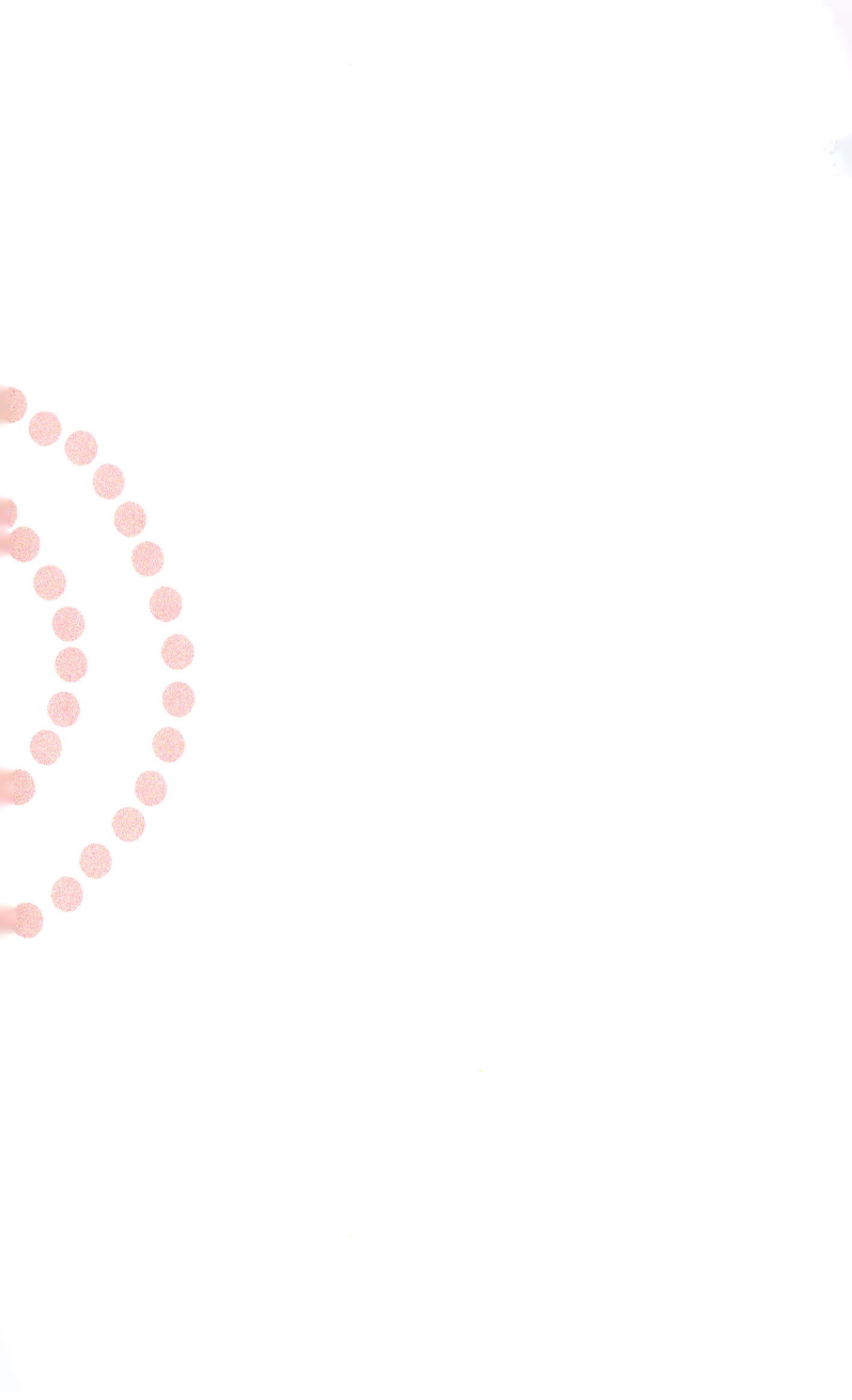

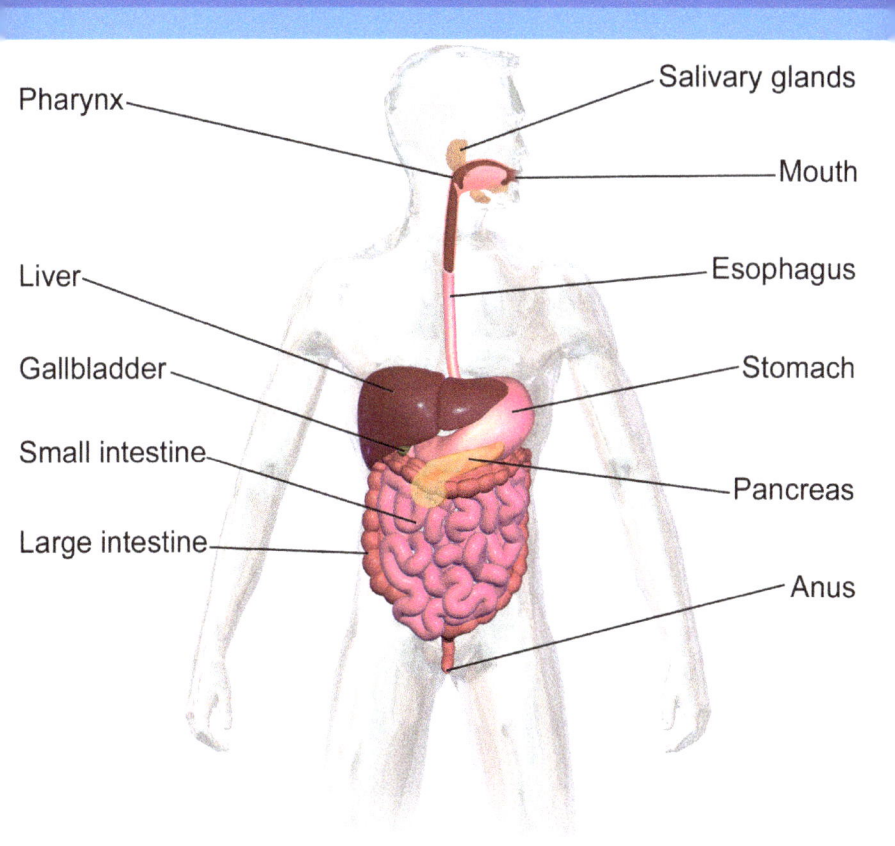

# THE ABDOMEN

**CHAPTER 8**

- Pharynx
- Salivary glands
- Mouth
- Liver
- Esophagus
- Gallbladder
- Stomach
- Small intestine
- Pancreas
- Large intestine
- Anus

Blausen.com staff (2014) "Medical gallery of Blausen Medical 2014 WikiJournal of medicine 1(2)

# ABDOMEN ISSUES

- **APPENDICITIS**
- **INTUSSUSCEPTION**
- **FUNCTIONAL ABDOMINAL PAIN**
- **CONSTIPATION**
- **DIARRHEA**
- **VOMITING**

## APPENDICITIS:

> Inflammation/infection of the appendix.
> Appendix is located in right lower corner of abdomen.

### SYMPTOMS:

- Vomiting.
- Fever.
- Abdominal pain that starts around the umbilicus and moves to the right lower corner of the abdomen over several hours.
- Pain is made worse with walking or jumping.
- Normally occurs in children older than 3 years of age .

### DIAGNOSIS AND TREATMENT:

- The medical provider will perform a physical examination.
- If available, an ultrasound of the abdomen can be diagnostic; if an ultrasound is not available, a CAT scan of the abodomen may be performed.
- Blood tests are performed.
- If appendicitis is suspected, the patient will be referred to a general surgeon.

## The Abdomen 87

### APPENDICITIS REQUIRES AN IMMEDIATE EVALUATION!

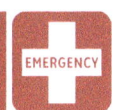

- Call your child's medical provider if the above symptoms develop during office hours.
- Go to the Emergency Room during non-office hours.

## INTUSSUSCEPTION:

Part of the small intestine telescopes inside neighboring intestine; does not normally involve the large intestine.
Can lead to an intestinal blockage.
Most common age group: 6 months to 3 years of age.

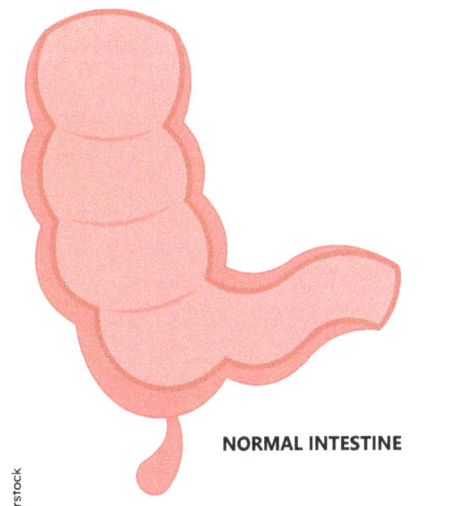

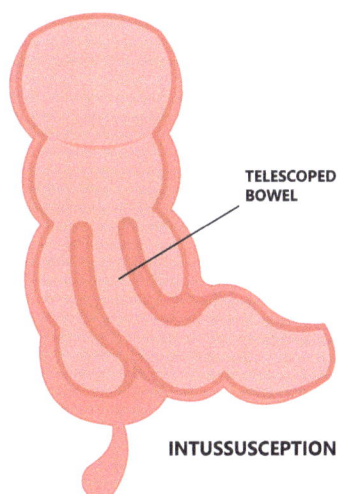

**NORMAL INTESTINE**

**INTUSSUSCEPTION**

TELESCOPED BOWEL

Pepermpron/Shutterstock

## CAUSES:

- It frequently occurs after a viral infection.

## SYMPTOMS:

- There is significant crampy abdominal pain that is usually intermittent (every 15 – 20 minutes) initially and then it becomes more constant.
- The child is usually very uncomfortable with the pain.
- The child may look pale and may be sweaty during the periods of pain.
- There can be red jelly looking stools passed as well.

### INTUSSUSCEPTION REQUIRES AN IMMEDIATE EVALUATION!

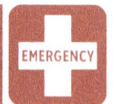

- **Call your child's medical provider if the above symptoms develop during office hours.**
- **Go to the Emergency Room during non-office hours.**

## DIAGNOSIS AND TREATMENT:

- Diagnosis is usually made by an ultrasound.
- Treatment consists of a contrast fluid enema performed by a pediatric radiologist to correct the intussusception.
- Very rarely is surgery needed.

# FUNCTIONAL ABDOMINAL PAIN:

> Abdominal pain that is recurring on a fairly regular frequency; typically occurs around the umbilical area; Usually occurs in children between 4- 16 years of age

## CAUSES:

- Not totally known yet.

## SYMPTOMS:

- Can have symptoms of vomiting, diarrhea, abdominal cramping or nausea.
- Not associated with fever.
- Can happen multiple times a month and it can vary as to the time of day it occurs.
- Usually has no relation to eating.
- Can occur (and often times it does) with stressful situations, for example – going to school.
- Normally does not wake the child during the night.
- Lab and xrays are always normal.
- The child continues to gain weight and grow in height.

## WHAT TO DO AT HOME:

- Consult with your child's medical provider.
- Be reassuring to your child during times of pain but yet try not to dwell on the abdominal pain.
- Encourage daily activities – staying active helps minimize the symptoms.

## DIAGNOSIS AND TREATMENT:

- The medical provider will take a detailed history and perform a physical exam.
- Additional work-up may include labs and possibly x-rays; the results are always normal in functional abdominal pain.
- The diagnosis is "one of exclusion" — functional abdominal pain is considered the probable diagnosis when physical exam and testing are all normal.
- There is not a specific medication to help eliminate this type of abdominal pain; there are some medicines available that your medical provider may prescribe to help with the symptom of abdominal pain.
- There is not a cure for it.

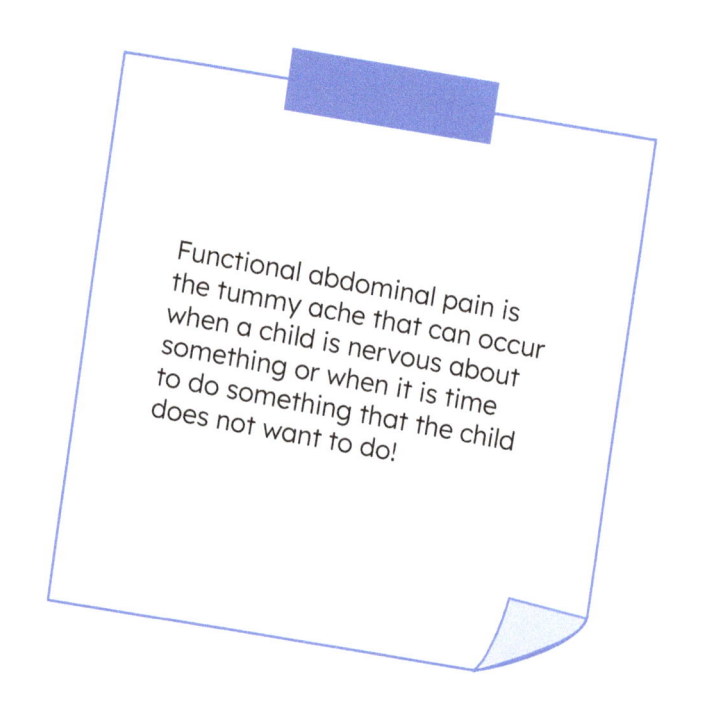

> Functional abdominal pain is the tummy ache that can occur when a child is nervous about something or when it is time to do something that the child does not want to do!

# CONSTIPATION:

> Quite common among infants, toddlers and children. Definition: constipation is the difficult passage of very firm hard stool or no stool at all.

## CAUSES:

- DIETARY:

    - Certain formulas for infants can cause firmer stools (soy in particular).
    - Lack of eating adequate fiber foods in toddlers and children.
    - Inadequate oral fluids during the day.
    - Excessive cow's milk.

- PURPOSEFUL HOLDING OF STOOL:

    - Common during "potty training".
    - Younger school age children hold stool during school hours because of not wanting "to go" at school. In addition, they delay toilet time because they do not want to stop what they are doing.

- PAINFUL PASSAGE OF STOOL:

    - Children will hold stool due to recent painful passage of stool out of fear that it will hurt again.

## WHAT TO DO AT HOME:

- To help "jump start" the passage of stool, give one dose of a children's laxative (see appendix for doses) OR insert a pediatric glycerin suppository into the child's rectum. If you cannot find a pediatric size, cut an adult suppository in half lengthwise. Cover the tip with some petroleum jelly (Vaseline®) to aid in insertion.

## The Abdomen

- Increase daily fluid intake.
- Can give 100% apple, pear or prune juice daily (4 oz) to help soften stool in anyone older than 4 months.
- Consider using Miralax® on a daily basis if the constipation is chronic; Miralax® is over the counter and very safe for toddlers and children (see Appendix for starting dose).
- Increase fiber content in the daily diet – (see Appendix for examples).
- DO NOT USE DARK KARO® SYRUP to treat infant constipation; it is no longer recommended because it does not contain the proper agent to draw water into the intestine (which is what helps soften the stool).

## DIAGNOSIS AND TREATMENT:

- Your child's provider will take a history of the problem and perform a physical exam.
- An x-ray of the abdomen may sometimes be required to diagnose the constipation – but it is not necessary in every case.
- Your child's provider may recommend a more intense plan of treating the constipation with medications.

  IMPORTANT: some breast fed infants can significantly decrease their stool output around one month of age. Several days can pass without any stool (up to one week!).
  When they do pass a stool, it is the typical loose, yellow and seedy breast fed stool.
  THIS IS NOT CONSIDERED CONSTIPATION!***

## WHEN TO CONTACT YOUR CHILD'S HEALTHCARE PROVIDER

- When the child is extremely uncomfortable with abdominal pain.
- When there has not been any stool for at least 4-5 days and the above measures have been taken.
- When there is bleeding associated with each stool passage.
- When the constipation is persistent.

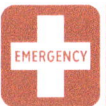

## WHEN TO GO TO THE EMERGENCY ROOM

- When the child is extremely uncomfortable with abdominal pain and your child's provider is not available.

---

Chronic constipation (constipation that lasts more than 3-4 weeks) is fairly common in children. Chronic constipation requires long term parental attention, supervision and treatment. Unfortunately, chronic constipation can take months to get under control.

# DIARRHEA:

Passage of loose, watery stools 3 or more times a day.

## CAUSES:

- INFECTION:

    - FROM A VIRUS
    - FROM BACTERIA
    - FROM A PARASITE

- ANTIBIOTIC THERAPY
- FOOD ALLERGY

# VIRAL DIARRHEA:

- This is the most common cause of diarrhea in infants and children.
- It is common to be associated with vomiting and sometimes abdominal cramping — this is called gastroenteritis (or the "stomach flu").
- Multiple viruses can cause gastroenteritis; this type of infection is usually quite contagious and can affect each family member.
- Usually lasts for several days in older children, and up to two weeks in younger children.

## WHAT TO LOOK FOR:

- In general, diarrhea by itself is less likely to cause dehydration in contrast to vomiting, however, excessive and frequent watery diarrhea can lead to dehydration on occasion. It is therefore important to monitor for dehydration in a child with diarrhea.
- Any significant abdominal pain.
- Number of stools in 24 hours.
- Any fever.
- Monitor for DEHYDRATION.

## The Abdomen

- WATCH URINE OUTPUT. Infants less than 6 months of age should have a wet diaper at least every 6 hours. Infants/children older than 6 months of age should have a wet diaper or urinate at least every 8 hours.
OTHER SIGNS OF DEHYDRATION:
    - Dry mouth, lack of saliva.
    - Decreased tears.
    - Sunken soft spot on the head of an infant.
    - Child is "limp as a dishrag"
    - Very fussy.
    - Extra sleepy.
    - Sunken eyes.
    - Cool hands and feet with purplish discoloration.

## WHAT TO DO AT HOME:

- Bland foods (toast, crackers, brothy soups, for example).
- Avoid spicy food, fatty food and dairy products until the diarrhea is improving.
- An age appropriate diet may restart once the child is drinking well.
- A "BRAT" diet was recommended in the past for treatment of diarrhea – it is now felt that this type of diet does not serve a purpose.
- Insure adequate fluid intake with: water, low sugar drinks, sports drinks, or home-made electrolyte fluid drinks (see Appendix for recipe). Try Pedialyte® for infants.
- **\*\* Do not give fruit juices.\*\***
- Currently, there is not good evidence from multiple studies that probiotics are of benefit in children with viral gastroenteritis.
- There are no medications recommended for the treatment of diarrhea in children younger than 8 years of age.
- \*\*Medications are discouraged for children older than 8 years of age for the treatment of diarrhea: it is felt that the potential side effects of medications that are used to slow down diarrhea outweigh the benefits.

## The Abdomen

### WHEN TO CALL YOUR CHILD'S PROVIDER OR GO TO THE EMERGENCY ROOM IF THE PROVIDER IS NOT AVAILABLE

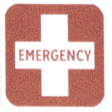

- **If there are any signs of dehydration.**
- **If urine output is less than above criteria.**
- **If your child is very uncomfortable with stomach pain.**
- **If number of stools per day exceeds 10.**
- **If fever persists beyond 24-48 hours.**
- **If there are more than 4 episodes of vomiting in 24 hours.**

### IMPORTANT:

- Good handwashing with soap and water can help prevent spread of viral gastroenteritis.
- Current recommendations from the Academy of Pediatrics for returning to daycare and/or school after a bout of diarrhea include:

    - Stools are contained in diaper.
    - Child does not have stooling accidents.
    - Stool frequency is less than 2 more than child's normal stool number per day.

- Even though this illness is sometimes called "the stomach flu", it has no relationship to Influenza ("the flu"). Each illness is caused by an unrelated virus and has very different symptoms.

- Do not give children a flour mixture to treat diarrhea.

## BACTERIAL DIARRHEA:
- Not as common as viral causes of diarrhea

## CAUSES:
- Common bacteria that cause this include E. Coli, Salmonella, Shigella, and Campylobacter.
- A common source of bacterial diarrhea is food that has not been prepared or stored correctly. For example, Campylobacter infection can come from under cooked chicken.

## SYMPTOMS:
- Associated symptoms can include fever, abdominal pain, vomiting and bloody diarrhea.

## WHAT TO LOOK FOR:
- Presence of bloody stools.
- Number of stools in 24 hours.
- Significan abdominal pain.
- Any fever.
- Frequency of vomiting.
- Monitor for DEHYDRATION:
  WATCH URINE OUTPUT. Infants less than 6 months of age should have a wet diaper at least every 6 hours. Infants/children older than 6 months of age should have a wet diaper or urinate at least every 8 hours.
  OTHER SIGNS OF DEHYDRATION:
    - Dry mouth, lack of saliva.
    - Decreased tears.
    - Sunken soft spot on the head of an infant.
    - Child is "limp as a dishrag"
    - Very fussy.
    - Extra sleepy.
    - Sunken eyes.
    - Cool hands and feet with purplish discoloration.

## WHAT TO DO AT HOME:

- Bland foods (toast, crackers, brothy soups, for example).
- Avoid spicy food, fatty food, and dairy products until diarrhea is improving.
- Age appropriate diet may restart once child is drinking well.
- A "BRAT" (Banana, Rice, Apple sauce, Toast) diet was recommended in the past for treatment of diarrhea – it is now felt that this type of diet does not serve a purpose.
- Insure adequate fluid intake with: water, low sugar drinks, sports drinks, home-made electrolyte fluid recipes (see Appendix for recipe) Pedialyte® for infants.
- **\*\* Do not give fruit juices.\*\***
- There are no medications for diarrhea in children younger than 8 years of age.
- \*\*Medications are discouraged for children older than 8 years of age with bacterial diarrhea: it is felt that the potential side effects of medications that are used to slow down diarrhea outweigh the benefits.

## WHEN TO CALL YOUR CHILD'S PROVIDER OR GO TO THE EMERGENCY ROOM IF THE PROVIDER IS NOT AVAILABLE

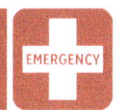

- **If urine output is less than above criteria.**
- **If your child is very uncomfortable with stomach pain.**
- **If number of stools per day exceeds 10.**
- **If there are more than 4 episodes of vomiting in 24 hours.**
- **If there are any signs of dehydration.**
- **If there is bloody diarrhea.**

## DIAGNOSIS AND TREATMENT:

- In order to diagnose a bacterial infection, samples of stool need to be sent to the lab for testing; results normally take at least 48 hours to come back.
- Depending on the bacteria that is found, antibiotics may be indicated. However, some bacterial infections go away on their own in otherwise healthy children and antibiotics are NOT recommended – in fact contraindicated.
- Probiotics have not been conclusively found to be indicated in bacterial diarrhea; some studies suggest that they may shorten the course of diarrhea by ½ to 2 days.

## IMPORTANT:

- Children may return to daycare/babysitter/school 24 hours after the last epidose of diarrhea from a bacterial infection.

## PARASITIC DIARRHEA:

### CAUSES:
- Common parasites: giardia, cryptosporidium.
- These types of infections are usually caused by drinking contaminated water – occasionally pool water, but more commonly from streams (cold mountain streams).
- Giardia is the most common parasitic infection causing diarrhea in the United States.

### SYMPTOMS:
- Similar to viral and bacterial diarrhea – but normally there is no bloody diarrhea.

### WHAT TO DO:
- Same instructions as for viral and bacterial diarrhea.

### DIAGNOSIS AND TREATMENT:
- To diagnose this type of infection, stool samples need to be sent to the lab.
- There are medications similar to antibiotics that can treat these infections.
- Probiotics have not been proven to be of significant benefit in this type of diarrhea in children.

### IMPORTANT:
- The child may return to daycare or school 24 hours after the last episode of diarrhea.

## DIARRHEA FROM ANTIBIOTIC THERAPY:

- We, as humans, have a population of bacteria, viruses and yeast that live harmlessly in our gut (the microbiome). They help with keeping bad versions of themselves from overtaking the gut and causing infection. They also help in digestion of complex sugars and fiber in the gut.
- When a person takes an antibiotic for whatever reason, the good bacteria living in the gut can be "killed" off by the antibiotic which then allows more problematic bacteria to grow in numbers and potentially lead to diarrhea.
- Normally, just stopping the antibiotic will help resolve the diarrhea.
- Some studies suggest that giving a probiotic in this type of diarrhea can be helpful in decreasing the number of days with diarrhea.
- An example of a more problematic bacteria that can be allowed to grow is called Clostridium Difficile. It is more common in older children and adults but can occasionally be found in younger children.
- This infection causes a very foul smelling stool – this is how it is sometimes suspected.
- If your child has been on a prolonged course of antibiotics, this may be a possibility. It is diagnosed with a stool sample sent to the lab. It is treated with a specific antibiotic.

## IMPORTANT:
- Having diarrhea as a side effect of taking an antibiotic is one of many reasons why it is important to not take an antibiotic unless there is a specific infection for which it has been prescribed by a medical provider.

## DIARRHEA FROM FOOD ALLERGY:

- Most gastrointestinal symptoms of a food allergy (vomiting and/or diarrhea) normally occur within two hours of consuming a food, and often they occur almost immediately. In very rare cases, the reaction can be delayed up to 6 hours after the ingestion of the food.
- Other symptoms of an allergy can also be present (vomiting, hives, fainting).
- The diarrhea is usually short-lived (it lasts less than 24 hours).

## WHAT TO DO:

- Give Benadryl® immediately (See dosage chart in Appendix).
- Contact your child's medical provider.

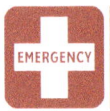

### WHEN TO CALL 911 OR GO TO THE EMERGENCY ROOM

- **CALL 911 if your child is having breathing difficulties and/or is lethargic.**
- **If there is any shortness of breath, generalized hives, swollen lips or tongue, go immediately to the nearest Emergency Room.**

- Once the acute allergic reaction has resolved, it will be important to follow up with your child's medical provider to verify the food allergy. This can be done by performing a blood test. If the food allergy is confirmed, your child will be prescribed an Epipen® (epinephrine autoinjector). This is to be used for any future allergic reactions. A Food Allergy Plan will also be provided to you; this is a written plan specific for your child that explains what treatment needs to be given at any future allergic reaction to food.

# VOMITING

## CAUSES:
- GASTROENTERITIS, a.k.a. "STOMACH FLU"
- GASTROESOPHAGEAL REFLUX (GERD)
- HEADACHES/MIGRAINE
- FOOD ALLERGIES
- PYLORIC STENOSIS

# GASTROENTERITIS:

> Fairly common and fairly contagious.
> Often will affect all family members over the course of several days.

## CAUSES:
- Caused by several families of viruses.

## SYMPTOMS:
- Starts with vomiting, then proceeds to diarrhea. The vomiting usually will resolve after 12-18 hours.
- Can be associated with abdominal pain and cramping.
- Fever may be present, but not always.

## WHAT TO DO AT HOME:
- Stop all regular foods until there has been no vomiting for 8 – 12 hours.
- Give small sips of hydrating fluids until there has been no vomiting for 8 – 12 hours. (see recipes for these fluids in the Appendix).

## WHAT TO DO AT HOME (continued):

- Advance foods slowly back into diet over next 1-2 days.
- Treat fever if present.
- With vomiting, it is very important to MONITOR FOR DEHYDRATION.
- WATCH URINE OUTPUT. Infants less than 6 months of age should have a wet diaper at least every 6 hours. Infants/children older than 6 months of age should have a wet diaper or urinate at least every 8 hours.

  OTHER SIGNS OF DEHYDRATION:
    - Dry mouth, lack of saliva.
    - Decreased tears.
    - Sunken soft spot on the head of an infant.
    - Child is "limp as a dishrag"
    - Very fussy.
    - Extra sleepy.
    - Sunken eyes.
    - Cool hands and feet with purplish discoloration.

  OBSERVE FOR OTHER SERIOUS SYMPTOMS:
    - Localized abdominal pain in right lower corner of abdomen.
    - Severe abdominal pain.
    - Bloody diarrhea.
    - Marked tiredness.
    - Bad headache.

## WHEN TO CALL YOUR CHILD'S PROVIDER OR GO TO THE E.R.

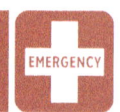

- **If any of the above serious symptoms or signs of dehydration are present, call your child's provider. If the provider is not available, go to the E.R.**

**ALSO, CALL YOUR CHILD'S PROVIDER IF VOMITING PERSISTS BEYOND 24 HOURS.**

## DIAGNOSIS AND TREATMENT:

- The medical provider will take a careful history and perform a physical exam to assess the child. Additionally, blood work may be performed to assess electrolyte abnormalities, dehydration, and other possible related conditions. If the child shows evidence of dehydration, the provider may refer him/her to a hospital for admission, or at least for IV fluids. If dehydration is mild or is not present, the child may return home to be managed with oral fluids. The provider may prescribe medications to treat the vomiting (Zofran® - ondansetron).

## IMPORTANT:

- There is not yet good evidence to support the use of probiotics with gastroenteritis.

# GASTROESOPHAGEAL REFLUX (GERD):

## IN INFANTS:

- Very common in all infants under the age of 9 months.
- Infants under 9 months of age do not have the mechanism that forces closure of the lower end of the esophagus after swallowing, therefore there is nothing that prevents contents of the stomach to re-enter the esophagus. This normally resolves around 9 months of age.
- There are no medicines that minimize or prevent reflux; an acid reducer is sometimes prescribed if an infant is exhibiting symptoms of painful "heartburn".
- Despite refluxing, spitting up, and vomiting, most infants continue to gain weight. If there is weight loss associated with reflux, referral to a pediatric gastroenterologist is recommended.
- There are no proven recommendations to help minimize the spit up/vomiting. Thickening formula, frequent burping, keeping the infant upright after feedings — these have all been suggested over the years, but it is questionable how successful those methods really are.
- Smaller, more frequent feedings may have some benefit in decreasing the amount of spit up.
- There are no long term side effects of reflux in infants.
- Reflux in infants is more of a nuisance for parents; the amount of laundry is increased, and parents and their clothes will often be on the receiving side of spit up.

## GERD - gastroesophageal reflux disease

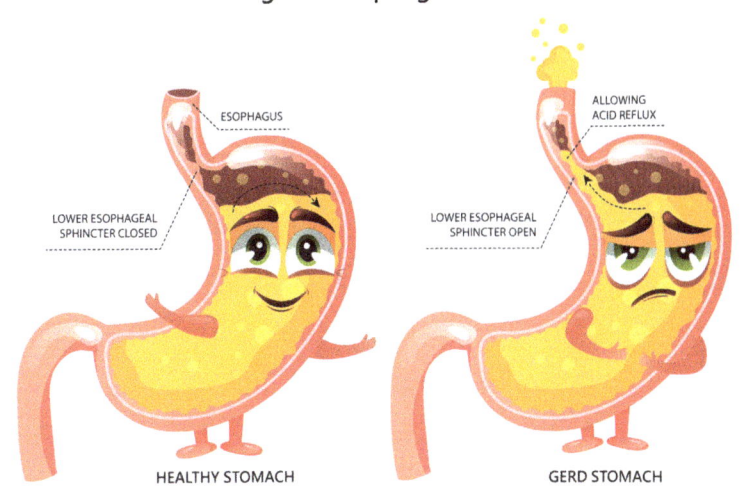

*HEALTHY STOMACH* — ESOPHAGUS, LOWER ESOPHAGEAL SPHINCTER CLOSED

*GERD STOMACH* — ALLOWING ACID REFLUX, LOWER ESOPHAGEAL SPHINCTER OPEN

# IN OLDER CHILDREN AND TEENAGERS:

- Reflux is not uncommon.
- Several factors that can lead to gastroesophageal reflux in this age group are:

  - Bed time snacks.
  - Snacking, eating within two hours of going to bed.
  - Drinking carbonated liquids (soda, flavored waters).
  - Drinking liquids containing caffeine (tea, coffee).

- Spit up/vomiting is not as common in older children as it is in infants with reflux.
- More common complaints of gastroesophageal reflux in children are:

  - Prolonged sore throat.
  - Hoarseness.
  - Cough.
  - Chest pain (heartburn).
  - Bad tast in mouth upon awakening in the morning.
  - Vomiting or waking up with abdominal pain during the night.

# DIAGNOSIS AND TREATMENT:

- The medical provider will take a careful history and perform a physical exam to determine the diagnosis. Blood tests may be done to rule out other conditions, but X-rays are not helpful in this situation. Only if symptoms persist, a gastroenterologist may perform a procedure looking directly at the esophagus (upper endoscopy).

- Lifestyle changes treatment options:
    - Minimize carbonated beverages.
    - Nothing to eat or drink for two hours before bedtime.
    - Decrease caffeine intake.
    - Elevate the head of the bed about 4 inches (place blocks under legs at head of bed).

- If there are symptoms of heartburn, an acid reducer can be taken for 2-3 weeks. Long term use of acid reducers in children is contraindicated (unless your child is seeing a GI doctor who is recommending it).

---

Reducing the risk of GERD is one of many good reasons to restrict soda intake in children and teenagers.

One 12 oz serving per week is a reasonable amount to allow.

## VOMITING CAUSED BY MIGRAINE HEADACHES:

- Vomiting is often associated with migraine headaches in children. The classic presentation of a childhood migraine headache is the rapid development of a headache, followed by vomiting usually within an hour. The child normally falls asleep after the vomiting, sleeps for a few hours and wakes up with much of the headache resolved.
- It is important to discuss these kinds of symptoms with your child's provider; if the headache resolves following a nap, it would not be necessary to go to an Emergency Room at that time. However, making an appointment for your child to be seen soon for evaluation would be recommended.
- IMPORTANT NOTE: If your child is having daily headaches associated with vomiting, it would be very important for your child to be seen by the child's provider promptly.

# VOMITING CAUSED BY FOOD ALLERGIES:

- Vomiting can be a symptom of a food allergy.
- It can occur within a few hours of a food being ingested.
- Occasionally there are other symptoms of an allergic reaction as well (hives, swelling of lips or tongue, shortness of breath and diarrhea).

## WHAT TO DO AT HOME:

- Give Benadryl® by mouth (dosages in appendix) immediately.
- Contact your child's healthcare provider.

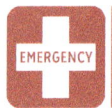

### WHEN TO CALL 911 OR GO TO THE EMERGENCY ROOM

- **CALL 911 if your child is having breathing difficulties and/or is lethargic.**
- **If there is any shortness of breath, generalized hives, swollen lips or tongue, go immediately to the nearest Emergency Room.**

- Once the acute allergic reaction has resolved, it will be important to follow up with your child's medical provider to verify the food allergy. This can be done by performing a blood test. If the food allergy is confirmed, your child will be prescribed an Epipen® (epinephrine autoinjector). This is to be used for any future allergic reactions. A Food Allergy Plan will also be provided to you; this is a written plan specific for your child that explains what treatment needs to be given at any future allergic reaction to food.

# PYLORIC STENOSIS:

A blockage at the outlet of the stomach, leading to projectile vomiting.
Classically, it occurs around one month of age in the first born male of the family; it can occur in female infants and subsequent siblings of the first born as well, but less often.

## CAUSE:

- The pylorus is a muscular valve at the junction of the stomach and small intestine; in some babies, this muscle thickens and does not allow stomach contents to empty into the small intestine. There is then a "back up" in the stomach of whatever the infant is drinking – leading to forceful or projectile vomiting after a feeding.

## SYMPTOMS:

- Projectile vomiting after EACH feeding.
- Infant acts hungry most of the time.
- Infant is fussier than normal.
- Possibility of decreased urine output secondary to the vomiting.

## WHAT TO DO AT HOME:

- Contact your child's healthcare provider.

## DIAGNOSIS AND TREATMENT:

- The healthcare provider will perform a physical examination of the infant after taking a careful history. The possibility of dehydration will be evaluated.
- An ultrasound of the abdomen is the diagnostic test that can easily be done to evaluate for pyloric stenosis

## 112 The Abdomen

- If pyloric stenosis is documented on ultrasound, the infant will be referred to a pediatric surgeon. The surgeon performs a surgical procedure cutting some of the thickened muscle of the pylorus, allowing the area to function normally again. Hospitalization for this is very short -term, usually 24 hours or less.
- The condition typically does not return.

### WHEN TO CONTACT YOUR CHILD'S HEALTHCARE PROVIDER

- **If your infant is between 3 and 5 weeks of age and projectile vomiting suddenly starts after every feeding.**

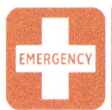

### WHEN TO GO TO THE EMERGENCY ROOM

- **If the situation above exists and you cannot contact your healthcare provider, go to an emergency room. (If at all possible, go to a children's hospital for care of this).**

# OTHER LESS COMMON REASONS FOR VOMITING:

- Motion sickness
- Extreme pain from another source, for example a kidney stone or kidney infection.
- There are treatment options for these conditions; contact your child's medical provider for recommendations.

# PINWORMS

## CAUSE:

- A tiny worm called Enterobius vermicularis; it looks like a ½ inch long piece of white thread.
- The eggs of pinworms are common in dirt; when ingested, they hatch into worms in the intestine
- This infection is common in toddlers and school age children. In addition to dirty hands and dirt under the fingernails, pinworm eggs can also be picked up from contaminated surfaces anywhere from toilet seats to bed clothes: when children put their fingers in their mouths, the eggs of pinworms are accidentally ingested and the infection starts.

## SYMPTOMS:

- Intense rectal itching shortly after going to bed (caused by the female worm coming out of the rectum at night to lay eggs).
- Sometimes the worms can be seen around the rectum during the time the child is itching at night (a bright flashlight helps to see them).
- The tiny worms can also be seen sometimes on the outside of stool.
- Girls may also have vaginal irritation due to the female worm migrating to the vagina from the rectum.

## WHAT CAN BE DONE AT HOME:

- If you strongly suspect pinworms, an over-the-counter treatment is available (pyrantel pamoate). It is strongly recommended that the entire family be treated at the same time because pinworm infections are highly contagious. Repeating the treatment in 2 weeks is also recommended.
- Instruct children to wash their hands thoroughly and often. Keep their fingernails short as well.
- Wash all exposed bed clothes, towels and clothing in hot, soapy water.
- Itching around the rectum may continue up to a week after treatment; over- the – counter hydrocortisone cream applied daily around the rectum can help with the itching.

## WHEN TO CONTACT YOUR CHILD'S HEALTHCARE PROVIDER

- **If symptoms persist after treating the infection with the over-the-counter medication, call your child's provider.**
- **There are prescription medications that can be prescribed as well for pinworm infections.**
- **If the diagnosis is questionable, the provider may order a stool test that can confirm the diagnosis.**
- **There are other conditions to consider if there are prolonged complaints of rectal and or vaginal itching or irritation, particularly if the complaints occur throughout the day.**

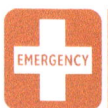

## WHEN TO GO TO THE EMERGENCY ROOM

- **Pinworm infections should not require an emergency room visit.**

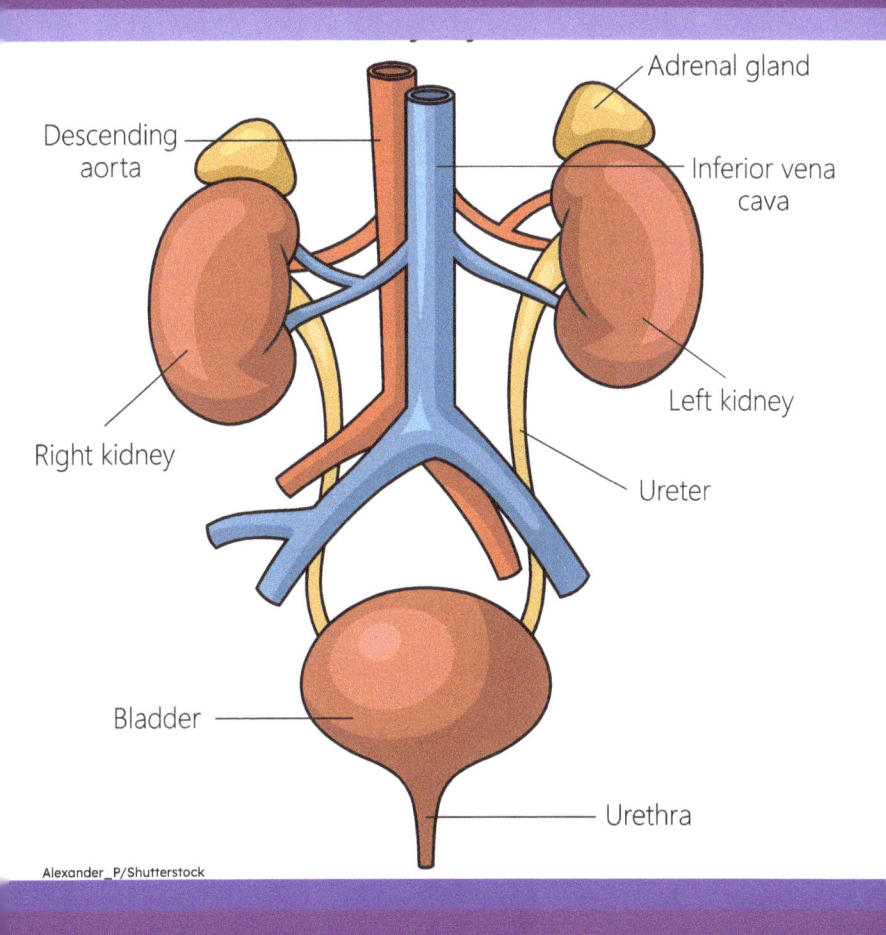

# THE GENITO URINARY SYSTEM

## CHAPTER 9

- Adrenal gland
- Descending aorta
- Inferior vena cava
- Right kidney
- Left kidney
- Ureter
- Bladder
- Urethra

# FEMALES:

CONDITIONS THAT ARE COMMON:
- Urinary Tract Infections (urination may be painful).
- Vulvovaginitis (urination may be painful).
- Vaginal discharge (no pain involved).
- Inguinal hernia.

# URINARY TRACT INFECTIONS:

- The most common form is an infection within the bladder (not involving the kidney).

## CAUSES:

- Introduction of bacteria from the rectal area into the urethra; this normally occurs from improper "wiping" in girls (back to front instead of the correct front to back).
- Infrequent urination.

## SYMPTOMS:

- Pain with urination.
- Frequency of urination.
- "Accidents" in underwear.
- New onset bedwetting.

## WHAT TO DO AT HOME:

- Push liquids.
- It is not recommended to give your child the "over-the-counter" medication for painful urination – the medication changes the urine to an orange color and makes the initial testing for a bladder infection very difficult.

## WHEN TO CONTACT YOUR CHILD'S HEALTHCARE PROVIDER

- When there are complaints of painful urination, frequent urination, "accidents", or new onset bedwetting.

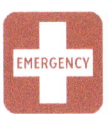

## WHEN TO GO TO THE EMERGENCY ROOM

- Only when you cannot contact your child's provider and your child is VERY uncomfortable with symptoms.

## DIAGNOSIS AND TREATMENT:

- At your medical provider's office, a urine sample is tested for immediate but preliminary results and it also is sent for culture (it is very important that the urine sample is a "clean catch" sample – your daughter's genital area is cleaned well first to wipe away any external contaminating germs before the actual urine is collected).

- If preliminary results of the urine testing suggest an infection, an antibiotic will be started; once culture results are known (in 48 hours), a final treatment decision will be made.

## PREVENTION:

- Remind your daughter to always wipe "front to back".
- Insure your child drinks adequate liquids throughout the day, every day.
- Insure that your child urinates at least every 4 hours during the awake day.

# VULVOVAGINITIS:

- This is a fairly common problem that consists of skin irritation in the area of the female genital labia; the most common age range is 3-8 yars of age.

## CAUSES:

- After successfully potty training, little girls suffer skin irritation from several sources:
    - Not wiping properly (either too much or too little).
    - Not rinsing the area well with water after using soap or bubble bath products in the bath tub water.
    - Wetting or leaking "accidents".
    - Infrequent cleaning of the genital area.

## SYMPTOMS:

- Redness of the labia on either side of the vaginal opening.
- Painful urination.
- An "odor".
- Itching.

## WHAT TO DO AT HOME:

- Insure proper cleaning of the external genital area on a daily basis.
- Always rinse the genital area with clean water after your daughter stands up out of the bath water (a squirt bottle works well for this).
- If there is redness of the area, apply petroleum jelly (Vaseline®), Aquaphor®, or A&D® ointment).

## WHEN TO CONTACT YOUR CHILD'S HEALTHCARE PROVIDER

- When the painful urination persists despite the above measures.

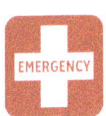

## WHEN TO GO TO THE EMERGENCY ROOM

- This condition should never require an Emergency Room visit.

## DIAGNOSIS AND TREATMENT:

- A physical examination is usually diagnostic.
- A "clean catch" urine sample may be obtained/evaluated.
- Symptomatic care is recommended (Vaseline®, Aquaphor® or A&D® ointment).

## IMPORTANT:

- Once past the age of 2 years, it is uncommon for girls to have genital yeast infections until after they start their periods.

# VAGINAL DISCHARGE:

- This is uncommon in girls until a year or two prior to starting their periods.

## CAUSES:

- A bacterial infection – most common type is a strep infection; but other bacteria could be the culprits.
- Foreign object in the vagina - little girls are capable of inserting small objects into their vaginal area, once the object is there for awhile, it can cause a discharge.
- "Pre"-period time.

## SYMPTOMS:

- Colored (yellow, green) vaginal discharge, may be tinged with blood.
- Occasionally an odor.
- Occasionally some redness of the skin around the vaginal opening.
- "Pre period" or early puberty discharge is usually clear to white and non-odorous. This is to be expected.

## WHAT TO DO AT HOME:

- Warm soaks in the bathtub.
- Application of petroleum jelly (Vaseline®), Aquaphor®, or A&D® ointment).

### WHEN TO CONTACT YOUR CHILD'S HEALTHCARE PROVIDER

- **Upon seeing any discolored (yellow, green or bloody) vaginal discharge, especially in a toddler or a child.**

## DIAGNOSIS AND TREATMENT:

- A history and physical examination by your child's provider.
- A sample of the vaginal discharge is sent for culture.
- Treatment will depend on the diagnosis/results of the vaginal culture.
- Removal of an object (if found) may need to be done by a Pediatric Gynecologist.

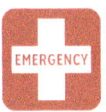

## WHEN TO GO TO THE EMERGENCY ROOM

- **A discolored vaginal discharge need not be seen in the Emergency Room.**
- **Keep in mind that your daughter may be much more comfortable seeing her own provider for this problem rather than a "stranger" provider elsewhere.**

---

It is important to teach your daughter, or son for that matter, at an early age (2 - 3 years of age) that there are limited people who have permission to look at or touch their genitalia.
Impress upon them to inform you if anyone who does not have permission makes an attempt to do so.

# INGUINAL HERNIA:

A visible bulge in the groin area; yes, girls can develop inguinal hernias.

## CAUSE:

- During fetal development, the inguinal canal, located between the lower abdomen and upper leg, is meant to close before birth. However, in some cases, it remains open, leading to an increased risk of inguinal hernias. This condition occurs when a portion of the intestines protrudes through an opening into the inguinal canal, potentially causing the ovary and Fallopian tube on the same side to fall into the hernia.

## SYMPTOMS:

- Usually appears as a bulge in the groin area.
- More obvious when the child is standing, crying, or bearing down. Usually disappears when the child lies down, stops crying, or is no longer bearing down.
- They usually are seen prior to age of 5 in girls; they are more common in premature infants.
- They are usually painless.

## WHAT TO DO AT HOME:

- There is no home treatment for a hernia.

### WHEN TO CONTACT YOUR CHILD'S HEALTHCARE PROVIDER

- **If you suspect that your child has a hernia, make an appointment with your child's medical provider. If there is no pain, no redness or other discoloration of the bulge, a non-emergent appointment would be appropriate.**

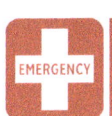

## WHEN TO GO TO THE EMERGENCY ROOM

> When you are unable to contact your child's provider, and there is swelling and redness.

## DIAGNOSIS AND TREATMENT:

- The provider will take a history and perform a physical examination.
- Normally, a hernia does not require additional testing for diagnosis.
- For an uncomplicated hernia, treatment is a non-emergent surgical repair performed by a general surgeon.
- For a hernia that is causing significant pain and distinct color changes of the bulge, an emergent surgical repair by a general surgeon is required.

# GIRLS GYNECOLOGY FACTS:

- Onset of periods (menarche) in girls can start in the general age range of 9-16 years.
- Periods normally start about 18 months after the initial appearance of coarse pubic hair.
- The pattern of periods in the first two years can be erratic or regular.
- Periods normally last 5-7 days.
- It is said that the frequency of periods is acceptable if they occur at least every 3 months and not more often than every 3 weeks.
- Bleeding with a period can be light or heavy. "Heavy" is described as needing to change a super absorbent pad or tampon at least once an hour. If your daughter does have heavy bleeding, contact her provider for further work up and care.
- Menstrual cramps do not normally start until roughly two years after periods have started. Ibuprofen is the drug of choice to use for cramps (as well as heavier bleeding in the first few days). One can start ibuprofen a day or two ahead of when the period should start to have better control of cramps and bleeding. If ibuprofen is not helping your daughter's cramps, contact her provider. There are other options that can be recommended.
- Tampons are an alternative to wearing sanitary napkins in girls; it is advisable that your daughter be mature enough to be able to insert the tampon as well as to remember to change it every 4-6 hours.
- For the daughter who has not yet started her periods, but is of the age, make sure that she has an "emergency kit" (sanitary napkin, clean underwear) in her backpack in the event that her period starts while she is at school or traveling.

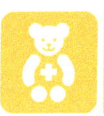

## WHEN TO CONTACT YOUR CHILD'S HEALTHCARE PROVIDER

- Your daughter is 16 and has not yet started her periods.
- If your daughter is having "heavy bleeding" as described above.
- If your daughter's menstrual cramps are not controlled with ibuprofen.
- If your daughter has started her periods and she is having periods more often than every 3 weeks or less often than every 3 months.

# MALES:

## PAINFUL SCROTUM:

### CAUSES:

- INFECTION

  - Viral.
  - Bacterial.
  - Involving the testis (Orchitis) or the epididymis (Epididymitis).

- BLOOD FLOW OBSTRUCION

  - Due to a twisting of the testis on its stalk – its blood supply (Torsion of the testis).
  - Due to a twisting of the appendage of the testis (Torsion of the testis appendage).

- TRAUMA

  - Usually due to a direct hit to the scrotum (contusion or hematoma).

### SYMPTOMS:

- Pain on affected side (can be very unfomfortable), swelling of the affected scrotal side, and redness of the scrotum.

### WHAT TO DO AT HOME:

- Attempt immediate pain control with ibuprofen or acetaminophen.

### WHEN TO CONTACT YOUR CHILD'S HEALTHCARE PROVIDER URGENTLY

- **Call your son's medical provider IMMEDIATELY if your son complains of pain in his scrotum and you see swelling or redness.**

## The Genito-Urinary System

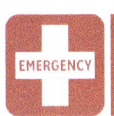

### WHEN TO GO TO THE EMERGENCY ROOM

- **When you are unable to contact your child's healthcare provider and there is swelling or redness of the scrotum.**

## DIAGNOSIS AND TREATMENT:

- A physical exam will be performed by your child's provider.
- A urine sample is normally checked.
- An ultrasound of the scrotum is very helpful in diagnosing the problem.
- If there is an infection diagnosed, the medical provider will prescribe an antibiotic.
- In the case of an infection, pain control with ibuprofen is recommended as are cool compresses laid over the scrotum. It will normally take 24-48 hours of treatment to give good pain relief.
- When an infection is present, it is recommended for the patient to wear tight underwear (not boxers) while this problem exists; the tight underwear give support to the scrotum, which will minimize pain.
- If the ultrasound confirms a torsion of the testis, an immediate referral to a pediatric urologist will be necessary. A torsion of the testis appendage does not require surgical intervention — it heals on its own.

## IMPORTANT:

- An infection can occur in either the testis or the epididymis. The typical age group for this to start is usually 14 years of age, but occasionally it can occur in younger boys.
- Torsion of the testis normally occurs in boys 10 years of age and older, but it can occur at an earlier age.

# HYDROCOELE:

- A fluid filled sac in the scrotum that surrounds the testis; it feels like a water balloon. There is no swelling above the scrotum (in contrast to an inguinal hernia).
- Normally seen in newborns and infants, but it can occur in children as well.
- Will sometimes appear as a pale blueish coloration under the skin of the scrotum.

## CAUSES:

- Not known.

## SYMPTOMS:

- This causes no significant pain/discomfort.
- This normally resolves on its own.

## WHAT TO DO AT HOME:

- No treatment is necessary.

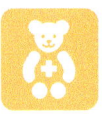

### WHEN TO CONTACT YOUR CHILD'S HEALTHCARE PROVIDER

- **Normally these are present at birth; the provider will point this out to you.**
- **Typically your child's provider will re-check this at each visit your infant has over the first several months of life.**

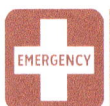

### WHEN TO GO TO THE EMERGENCY ROOM

- **A visit to the Emergency Room would not be necessary for this condition.**

# The Genito-Urinary System 129

## DIAGNOSIS AND TREATMENT:
- Normally this condition is self-evident to the provider.
- Rarely would an ultrasound be necessary.
- Treatment is usually observation.
- Hydrocoeles resolve on their own a majority of the time; if one seems to be increasing in size and/or the time span for one to resolve has passed, referral to a urologist may be necessary.

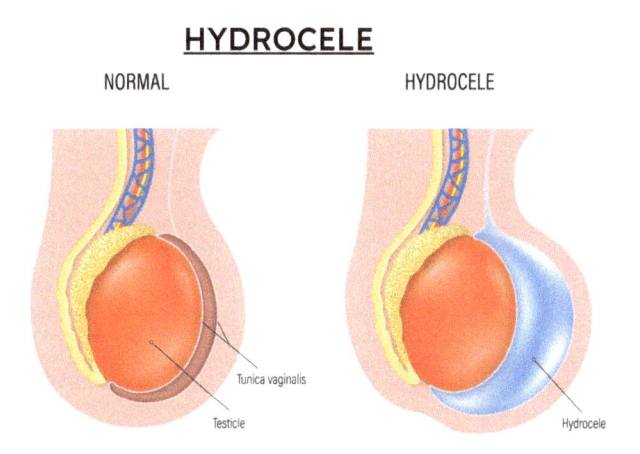

### HYDROCELE

NORMAL — HYDROCELE

*Labels: Tunica vaginalis, Testicle, Hydrocele*

### VARICOCELE

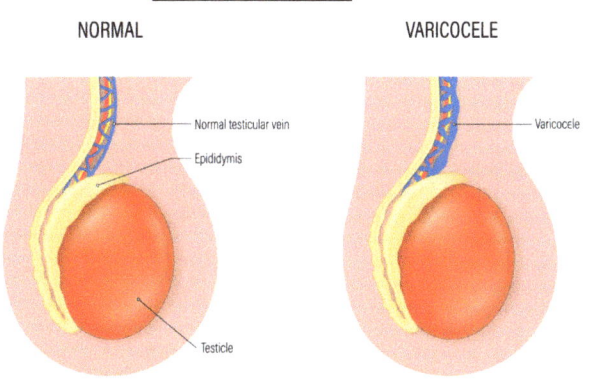

NORMAL — VARICOCELE

*Labels: Normal testicular vein, Epididymis, Testicle, Varicocele*

# VARICOCOELE:

- A "varicose vein" of the left testicular vein; this only occurs on the left side of the scrotum.

## CAUSE:

- Increased hydrostatic pressure in the testicular vein due to its anatomy.

## SYMPTOMS:

- Typically painless.
- Normally, it is evident as a soft "mass" located above the left testis (usually smaller than the testis itself).

### WHEN TO CONTACT YOUR CHILD'S HEALTHCARE PROVIDER

- **On a non-emergent basis; just to have it checked out.**

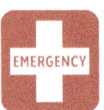

### WHEN TO GO TO THE EMERGENCY ROOM

- **A visit to the Emergency Room would not be necessary for this condition.**

## DIAGNOSIS AND TREATMENT:

- Your child's medical provider will perform a physical exam.
- An ultrasound is very helpful to confirm the diagnosis.
- No treatment is usually necessary; if it is causing pain, a referral to a urologist is made. Surgery is sometimes performed.

## IMPORTANT:

- Occurs in about 15% of males.
- Normally appears between 15 – 25 years of age.

# HERNIA (INGUINAL):

- A visible bulge in the groin area or the scrotum.

## CAUSES:

- During time in the womb, the testicles descend down from the abdominal cavity, through the inguinal canal (located in the crease between the lower abdomen and upper leg), and then into the scrotum. The pathway from the abdomen into the inguinal canal sometimes does not close prior to birth, as it should. This allows part of the intestines from the abdominal cavity to slip into the inguinal canal and then possibly the scrotum.

## SYMPTOMS:

- Usually painless.
- Usually appears as a bulge in the groin and possibly into the scrotum.
- More obvious when the child is standing, crying, or bearing down.
- Usually disappears when the child lies down, stops crying, or is no longer bearing down.

## WHAT TO DO AT HOME:

- There is no specific treatment that needs/can be done for a hernia at home.

### WHEN TO CONTACT YOUR CHILD'S HEALTHCARE PROVIDER

- **If you suspect that your child has a hernia, make an appointment with your child's provider. If there is no pain, redness, or other discoloration of the scrotum, this does not need to be done emergently.**

## WHEN TO CONTACT YOUR CHILD'S MEDICAL HEALTHCARE URGENTLY

- When the hernia is causing pain and/or there is red discoloration of the skin overlying the hernia.

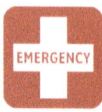

## WHEN TO GO TO THE EMERGENCY ROOM

- When you are unable to contact your child's healthcare provider and the hernia is causing pain and/or there is red discoloration of the skin overlying the hernia.

## DIAGNOSIS AND TREATMENT:

- The provider will take a history and perform a physical examination.
- Normally, a hernia does not require additional testing for diagnosis.
- For an uncomplicated hernia, treatment is a non-emergent surgical repair performed by a general surgeon.
- For a hernia that is causing significant pain and distinct color changes of the scrotum, an emergent surgical repair performed by a general surgeon may be required.

# BEDWETTING (NOCTURNAL ENEURESIS)

> Fairly common through the first 5 – 6 years of age; some children do not outgrow it until early teen years. Experts suggest that 15-20 percent of 5 year olds are still bedwetting and 10 percent of 7 year olds are still bedwetting at least parttime.
> It is more common in boys.
> There is a relatively strong family history associated with bedwetting.

## CAUSES:

- Internal control of bedwetting develops over time: sooner in some children, later in others.

## WHAT TO DO:

- Restrict fluids after 6 pm.
- Make sure your child empties his/her bladder before going to bed.
- Consult your child's medical provider after 6 years of age.

## TREATMENT:

- There are several options in the quest to treat bedwetting; success rates vary from child to child and from medication to medication:

  - DDAVP - this is a prescription medication taken at bedtime; it is helpful in about 50 % of children who take it;
  - Ditropan – this is a prescription medication; it usually works initially, but its effect starts to lessen over time;
  - Alarms – these are worn on the pajamas and set off an alarm as they sense wetness on the clothing. These may work for a while, but the child often becomes less responsive to the alarm over time.
  - Time – bedwetting does eventually resolve - it is just a matter of when.

## IMPORTANT:

- Be practical! Have a mattress protector on your child's bed.
- Allow your child to wear a pull-up if desired, wearing one does not delay resolution of bedwetting.
- Have your child help you with the washing of the bedclothes when they require washing.
- Do not punish your child for wetting the bed: it is not an intentional act!

# CHAPTER 10
# THE EXTREMITIES

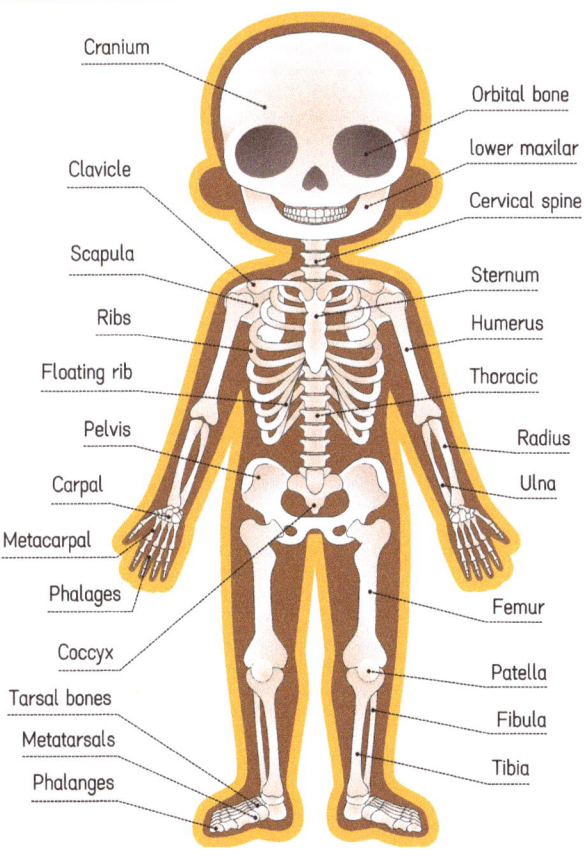

- Cranium
- Orbital bone
- lower maxilar
- Clavicle
- Cervical spine
- Scapula
- Sternum
- Ribs
- Humerus
- Floating rib
- Thoracic
- Pelvis
- Radius
- Carpal
- Ulna
- Metacarpal
- Phalages
- Coccyx
- Femur
- Patella
- Tarsal bones
- Fibula
- Metatarsals
- Tibia
- Phalanges

creekpan/Shutterstock

# EXTREMITIES

PROBLEMS:

- **GROWING PAINS**

- **JOINT PAIN**
    - **Post viral inflammation of the joint**
    - **Specific hip problems**
    - **"Overuse" syndrome**
        - Osgood-Schlatter disease
        - Chondromalacia patella
        - Heel pain

- **INJURIES**
    - **Fractures**
    - **Sprains/Strains**
    - **Nursemaid elbow**
    - **Foot pain**

# GROWING PAINS:

- Common in the age range of 3-12 years.
- Occurs in both boys and girls.
- The cause is unknown.
- Pain is usually in the long bones of the arms and legs – does not involve the joints.
- They occur on both sides of the body (maybe not at the same time). They do not affect just the same isolated extremity each time.
- They usually occur later in the evening or during the night.
- They may wake the child during the night.
- Growing pains are not serious.

## WHAT TO DO:
- Massage or rub the area that hurts.
- Give your child acetaminophen or ibuprofen for the pain.

### WHEN TO CONTACT YOUR CHILD'S HEALTHCARE PROVIDER
- **Pain is only in the same extremity each time.**
- **Pain in the extremity occurs during the day.**
- **When your child is favoring the extremity or not using it.**

# JOINT PAIN:

- In children, there are several conditions that can lead to joint pain. The majority are not serious and resolve over a short time.
- Rheumatoid disease in children is fairly rare and this will not be discussed in this book.

## POST-VIRAL INFLAMMATION OF THE JOINT:

- Not associated with fever; the joint pain normally comes after the fever leaves.
- There can be swelling of the joint, but normally there is no redness or warmth of the joint.
- Typically, the child will still move the joint – it is just somewhat painful.
- The pain usually will last for a few days and then resolve.
- The pain can be treated with ibuprofen.
- Joint pain usually occurs <u>after</u> a viral illness such as a cold, or a febrile illness.

### WHEN TO CONTACT YOUR CHILD'S HEALTHCARE PROVIDER

- **When your child will not walk due to the pain in the hip, knee or ankle.**
- **When your child will not use an arm due to pain in the elbow or wrist.**
- <u>**When there is generalized fever and redness/warmth in the joint.**</u>

# SPECIFIC HIP PROBLEMS:

▸ There are three specific conditions to know about:

### Toxic synovitis of the hip:
- Usually follows a viral illness.
- Occurs more often in 3-8 year-old boys.
- Usually occurs only on one side.
- Is usually treated with rest and ibuprofen.
- Usually resolves over 3 – 7 days.

### Avascular necrosis of the hip (Legg-Calve-Perthes disease):
- Usually presents with pain in the hip, thigh, or knee.
- Usually occurs in 4 – 10 year olds.
- Onset of pain (or limp) is very slow and over a long period of time.
- Diagnosis is by physical exam and xrays.
- Requires an orthopedic consultation.

### Slipped Capital Femoral Epiphysics (SCFE)
- Usually presents with pain in the hip, thigh or knee.
- Occurs more often in 12-14 year-old boys.
- Pain develops over a few weeks.
- Diagnosis is by physical exam and xrays.
- Requires an orthopedic consultation.

\*\* In any situation involving a limp, observation is acceptable for 1-2 days, provided that there is no fever. If the limp is resolving, the child can be watched at home. If the limp persists or lasts for more than 2-3 days, contact your child's provider. A limp would not require an emergency room visit normally, unless directed to do so.

\*\* If there is a fever associated with a limp, call your healthcare provider for an urgent appointment.

# OVERUSE SYNDROMES:

## OSGOOD-SCHLATTER DISEASE:

Besides the knee pain, the other most notable finding on exam is the "bump" that develops just below the knee cap, on one or both legs. The constant tugging and pulling of the patellar tendon on the area of bone just below the knee where the tendon attaches leads to inflammation and the formation of the bump. It tends to develop in the more rapid growth phase of children, as they enter puberty. It is more common in boys (but does occur in girls) who are active and is commonly seen in 10 - 15 year olds.

### WHAT CAN BE DONE AT HOME:

- Ice packs to the pain area.
- Ibuprofen or other anti-inflammatory pain medication as needed.
- Reduce sports activities when the pain is bothersome.
- Exercises specific for this condition.

### DIAGNOSIS:

- A physical exam performed by your child's healthcare provider or an orthopedist can confirm the diagnosis.
- X-rays are occasionally performed.

## CHONDROMALACIA PATELLA:

The knee pain associated with this is primarily around the kneecap. There is no swelling associated with this condition. The pain is dull and achey. It can involve just one or both knees. The underneath surface of the patella (knee cap) becomes inflamed from rubbing on the bones underneath it and it leads to pain. The pain is intensified by climbing stairs, sitting for a while, squatting, and running. This is more common in teenage females, but can occur in teen males.

### WHAT CAN BE DONE AT HOME:

- Ice packs to the affected knee.
- Excercises to strenghten the quadricep muscles.
- Ibuprofen or other anti-inflammatory pain medication as needed.

### DIAGNOSIS:

- A physical exam performed by your child's healthcare provider or an orthopedist can confirm the diagnosis.
- X-rays are occasionally performed to rule out other conditions, but they are not necessary to make the diagnosis.

## HEEL PAIN:

- Usually occurs between 8 and 14 years of age.
- Pain is from irritation of the growth area of the heel.
- Pain usually occurs after activity, and it is usually aggravated by activities with lots of running.
- Also known as Sever's disease.
- Child may continue to play sports as tolerated.

**WHAT CAN BE DONE AT HOME:**

- When pain occurs, treat with ice pack for 20-30 minute intervals.
- May use ibuprofen for pain.
- Heel cups worn in all shoes can be helpful, especially in sports' shoes. Heel cups may be purchased online or at most major drugstores.
- Calf stretches also help.

### WHEN TO CONTACT YOUR CHILD'S HEALTHCARE PROVIDER

- **For confirmation of the diagnosis.**
- **When pain is persisting despite treatment.**

# INJURIES:

## FRACTURES:
- Commonly due to falls and bike wrecks.

## CAUSES:
- In a child, one of the most common places for a fracture to occur is the arm (wrist and just above elbow area); it happens as the child puts out his hand to catch himself while falling.

## WHAT TO DO:
- Go to the ER with any obvious deformity.
- DO NOT give any pain medicine in case the child will require anesthesia to care for the fracture.
- If possible, try to provide support to the extremity that is injured and attempt to keep it elevated.
- Apply an ice pack to the area of injury to help reduce swelling.
- If there is not an obvious deformity, immobilizing and icing the injured area and treating pain as necessary, can safely be done until you can contact your child's provider for more direction.

## SPRAINS AND STRAINS:

- **TO CLARIFY**: a SPRAIN is an injury to a ligament(s) of a joint; a STRAIN is an injury to muscles and tendons (usually from being stretched). Bruising can occur with a sprain; it will not normally occur with a strain.

- ANKLE SPRAINS:
    - Most common type of sprain in chidren.
    - Commonly occurs when one "rolls" their ankle.
    - The swelling normally occurs on the outside of the ankle and can be impressive, at times.

- WRIST, FINGER AND KNEE SPRAINS:
    - Less common than ankle injuries.
    - They are often sports related injuries.

## WHAT TO DO AT HOME:

- Recommendations are fairly specific: "RICE"

    R = Rest: try to give the injury 24-48 hours of rest.

    I = Ice: ice the area injured for 20-30 minutes every 2 hours for the first day and 3-4 times a day over the next several days after injury. DO NOT put ice directly on the skin – wrap the bag containing ice in a towel before putting it over the injured area.

    C = Compression – wrap the involved area with an Ace wrap to minimize swelling and provide support. DO NOT make it too tight.

    E = Elevate – keep the injured area elevated (ideally at or above the level of the heart) for the first 24-48 hours to minimize swelling.

- Give ibuprofen for pain (usually works better than acetaminophen in this situation).

## WHEN TO CALL YOUR CHILD'S PROVIDER OR GO TO THE EMERGENCY ROOM IF THE PROVIDER IS NOT AVAILABLE

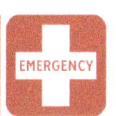

- When there is an obvious deformity of the joint.
- When your child cannot put any weight on the injured lower extremity
- When your child cannot use the injured upper extremity at all.

---

### TRAMPOLINE SAFETY

Trampolines are a favorite of children to play on - but they are the cause of numerous injuries – including fractures, strains and sprains. Head and neck injuries also occur on a trampoline.

Pediatricians discourage children playing on trampolines because of the high risk of injuries. But, if your family has a trampoline, here are some guidelines to follow to minimize injuries:

- No one under 6 years of age should jump on a trampoline.
- Only one child should jump at a time.
- No flips or somersaults should be allowed.
- A responsible adult should always supervise children on a trampoline.
- Jump only in the center.
- A net around the trampoline must be in place and secure.
- If the springs of the trampoline cannot be outside the net, they must be padded.
- No other objects should be on the trampoline or being held by someone while jumping.

## NURSEMAID'S ELBOW:

- Typically occurs in toddlers and children under 6 years of age.

## CAUSES:

- Usually occurs suddenly during a time when a toddler/child is holding hands with another person and is resisting and/or pulling away from that other person.
- The toddler/child suddenly starts crying holding his/her arm. Sometimes the other person can hear a "pop".
- When the injury occurs the ligament that holds the radius in place at the elbow joint slips and the end of the radius shifts out of position.

## SYMPTOMS:

- The child is uncomfortable/crying.
- Typically the child is holding the affected arm still at his/her side and does not want to bend it at the elbow.

## WHAT TO DO AT HOME:

- Unless you have been instructed by a physician how to "fix" the problem, do not make any attempt to fix it.
- You can give pain relief in the form of acetaminophen or ibuprofen (see dosages in appendix).

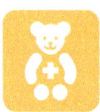

### WHEN TO CONTACT YOUR CHILD'S HEALTHCARE PROVIDER

- **Within 24 hours of the injury if your child is still complaining and not wanting to use the involved arm.**

## The Extremities 147

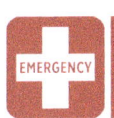

### WHEN TO GO TO THE EMERGENCY ROOM

> **If your child is crying or is uncomfortable and you are unable to contact your provider for recommendations.**

## DIAGNOSIS AND TREATMENT:

- With getting a history of the accident and a physical exam, a pediatrician will often treat the problem without getting an x-ray.
- A fairly simple maneuver can treat the problem.
- The provider feels a "pop" in the elbow as the elbow is maneuvered to fix the problem.
- The child will ypically start using the arm normally again quickly thereafter.
- Only if the child still refuses to use the arm after the treatment and/or is still in pain, is an x-ray obtained.
- If seen by a provider who is not familiar with Nursemaid's Elbow, an Xray is typically ordered first.
- The xray is normal in the case of Nursemaid's Elbow.

## IMPORTANT:

- Often, this injury can recur in toddlers and young children that have experienced at least one prior episode.
- In these children, one wants to avoid holding them by the hand, picking them up by their hands – anything that potentially straightens the elbow out leading to displacement of the ligament again.
- Children outgrow this potential problem by age 6 years.

# FOOT PAIN:

- In addition to obvious trauma that can lead to foot pain and possibly fractures in the foot, there are other possibilities that need to be considered in children (in the absence of trauma). They are:

  - A foreign object in the bottom of the foot that the child could have stepped on while barefoot – for example, a splinter, a piece of glass).
  - A plantar wart (discussed under Skin).
  - A bruise to the bottom of the foot.
  - Shoes too tight (with as quickly as children grow, this is not uncommon).
  - A stress fracture (more common in children above the age of 10)

## WHAT CAN BE DONE AT HOME:

- Look at the bottom of the foot and see if you see anything obvious.
- Try to remove a superficial splinter or other object if you can.
- A plantar wart can be treated with OTC medications (see more information in the Skin section).
- Check out the shoes your child has been wearing for proper size or any other issues with the shoe.

## WHEN TO CONTACT YOUR CHILD'S HEALTHCARE PROVIDER

- **If your child is consistently limping and/or there is a known injury that occurred.**
- **If it appears that there is a foreign object in the foot that you cannot successfully remove.**

# THE SKIN
## CHAPTER 11

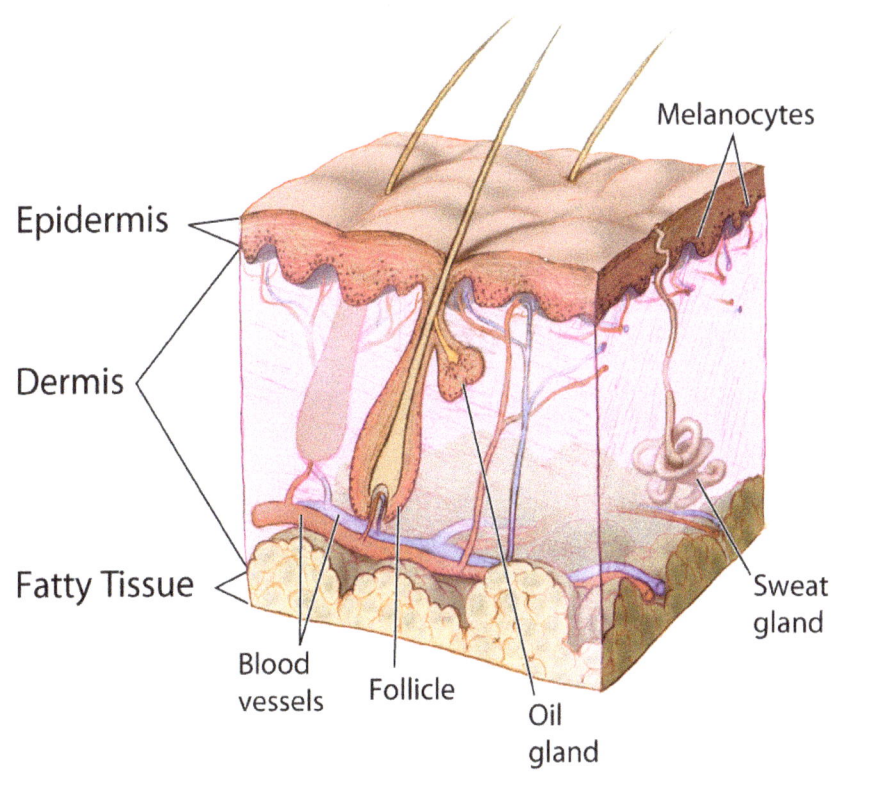

149

- Epidermis
- Dermis
- Fatty Tissue
- Blood vessels
- Follicle
- Oil gland
- Melanocytes
- Sweat gland

Don Bliss (artist), Public domain, via Wikimedia Commons

# RASHES

- Rashes are very common in infants and children; they come in different forms and different age groups.

- Some of them itch, some of them don't. Some are serious, the majority are not.

- There are many different conditions that can cause a rash. This section hopefully helps with identifying which rash your child has.

- The rashes have been grouped according to their general characteristic: bumpy, flat (or almost flat), flaky (scaly, crusty).

# RASHES THAT ARE BUMPS:

## CHICKENPOX (VARICELLA):

- Normally start as small red bumps (1/4 inch in diameter) scattered over the body; within 24 hours, the red bumps have developed a blister on top. Over the course of the next 1-2 days, the blisters then pop and scabs form.

- More chicken pox "spots" can erupt over the first 5-6 days so one can have chicken pox lesions in various stages.

- Lesions can occur anywhere on the body (they are normally equally spread out over the body) and inside the mouth. Lesions go away completely by 14 days after appearance; a child may have a few "scars" (little indents in the skin) that are permanent.

**The Skin 151**

CHICKEN POX/VARICELLA rash

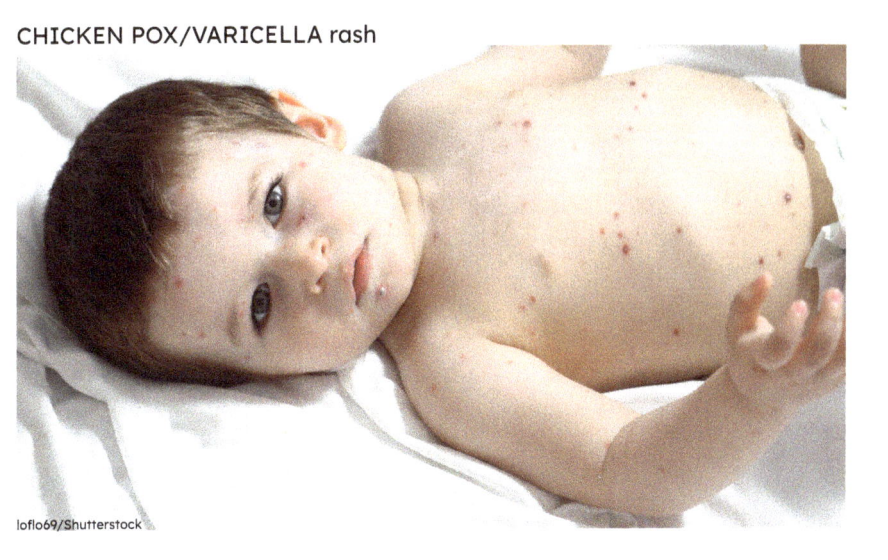

## SYMPTOMS:

- Some fever (maybe low grade or fairly high) and the child may not feel well.

- Chickenpox lesions can itch and there may be a sore throat or sore mouth if there are spots in the mouth.

- Child may complain of a headache.

- Normally there are no cold symptoms, vomiting/diarrhea.

## TREATMENT:

- Anti-itch medication (Benadryl® or longer acting anti histamine) for the itching.

- Fever control with acetaminophen or ibuprofen (see dosage chart in appendage).

- DO NOT give aspirin during this illness!

- The actual sores do not need treatment.

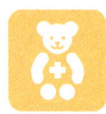

## WHEN TO CONTACT YOUR CHILD'S HEALTHCARE PROVIDER

- **If you think your child has chicken pox, call your child's medical provider.**
- **Verification needs to be done (there are lab tests that can be done to verify the diagnosis).**
- **Chicken pox is now a reportable condition to the Health Department, so it needs to be confirmed.**

## HOW LONG IS THE CHILD CONTAGIOUS:

- Incubation period (time from exposure to breaking out) is 3–7 days.
- Child is contagious from 24 hours before the first appearance of "spots" until all sores are scabbed over (usually 7-10 days after breakout).
- It is very important for a child with chicken pox to isolate at home and not attend school, daycare, or a babysitter's.

## ADDITIONAL INFORMATION:

- This infection has significantly decreased in the United States and the civilized world due to the introduction of the chicken pox vaccine in 1987. It is very rare for immunized children older than one year of age to develop chicken pox. Occasionally, an infant under one year of age may get chicken pox if they are exposed to someone who has shingles. Shingles is also caused by the chicken pox virus and can occur in a person who has had chicken pox in the past or in anyone who has had the chicken pox vaccine. Chicken pox in a healthy child is usually a mild illness and is well tolerated. However, if a child's immune system is compromised due to chemotherapy or other reasons, chicken pox can be a very serious illness. In such cases, it is important to contact a healthcare provider immediately.

**The Skin** 153

# CONTACT DERMATITIS:

## CAUSE:
- An allergic reaction in the skin caused by several substances – certain metals (in jewelry, belt buckles, clothing snaps), perfumes, cosmetics, and plants.
- The plant oils of poison ivy, poison oak and poison sumac cause allergic reactions in the top layers of the skin upon contact.
- The rash may appear within 12 hours or take up to 5 days after exposure.

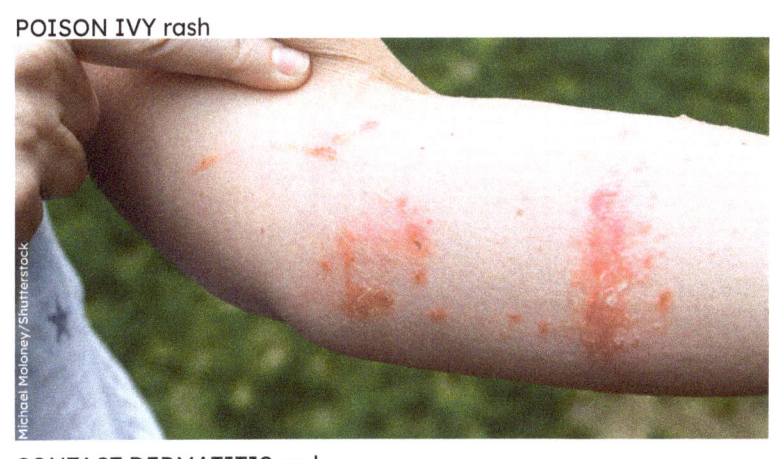

POISON IVY rash

CONTACT DERMATITIS rash

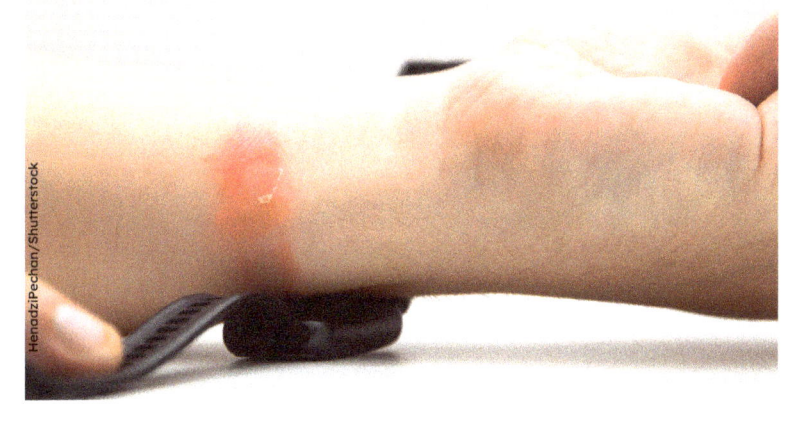

## SYMPTOMS:

- The rash is usually very itchy – it can sometimes burn as well.
- The rash is usually raised, red, and blistery.
- The rash of poison ivy, poison oak, and poison sumac can be linear, in groupings, or wide-spread depending on the pattern of exposure to the plant oil.
- People sometimes confuse shingles with poison ivy due to the similarities in appearance of the two rashes.

## WHAT TO DO AT HOME:

- Treat the itching with a short acting (Benadryl®) or long acting antihistamine (Zyrtec®, Claritin®).
- Cool wet compresses laid on the rash can be soothing and help with itching.
- Application of OTC steroid cream (1% hydrocortsone cream) can be helpful.
- The rashes caused by any of the above mentioned substances are not contagious.
- When a known exposure, especially to a plant, has occurred, wash the area as soon as possible with cool water and soap.
- Be careful when taking off clothing that may have been in contact with a plant – the plant oil on the clothing may come in contact with the skin and still cause a rash. In addition, it is important to wash any clothing exposed to the plant in hot, soapy water.

## WHEN TO CONTACT YOUR CHILD'S HEALTHCARE PROVIDER

- **It is advisable to contact your child's healthcare provider if the rash is widespread and/or if it is extremely itchy, preventing your child from sleeping or relaxing**

## DIAGNOSIS AND TREATMENT:

- Diagnosis can easily be made by the provider with just visual inspection of the rash
- Your child's provider may prescribe a prescription strength steroid cream to apply to the rash and in some cases, may prescribe an oral steroid, depending on the severity of the rash.

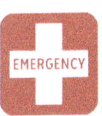

## WHEN TO GO TO THE EMERGENCY ROOM

- **Normally, it would not be necessary to be seen in the Emergency Room with this condition.**
- **Contact your child's provider first to get recommendations.**

## IMPORTANT POINTS:

- Again, be careful when taking off clothing that may have been in contact with a plant – the plant oil on the clothing may come in contact with the skin and still cause a rash.
- Family pets who go outside can potentially come in contact with the plants of poison ivy, poison sumac, and poison oak. The plant oil will attach itself to the animal's fur. If your child comes in contact with the pet's fur, the oil then contacts the skin and can cause the rash.
- Burning wood that has the plant of poison ivy, sumac or oak on it can cause the oil to be dispersed in the smoke of the fire. Anyone allergic to one of the plants who is in contact with the smoke can break out in the rash on all exposed skin.

# 156 The Skin

## PREVENTION:

- Avoid wearing known jewelry that causes rashes; snaps on clothing can be covered over to help prevent a rash.
If one is allergic to certain plants, either avoid them at all cost or wear long sleeved shirts and long pants when contact is possible. Wash all exposed skin as soon as possible.

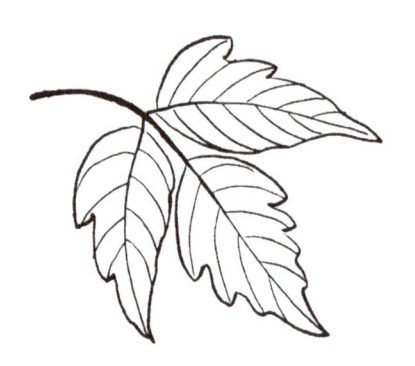

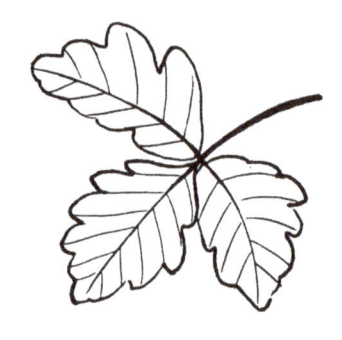

**poison ivy**

**poison oak**

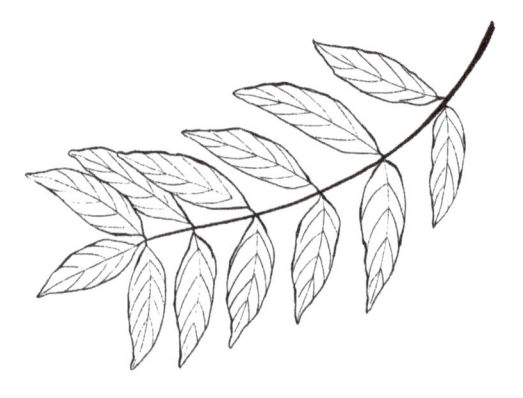

**poison sumac**

# HAND, FOOT, AND MOUTH DISEASE:

## CAUSE:

- Is caused by Coxsackievirus A16 most of the time; there are other Coxsackie viruses that can cause it as well.

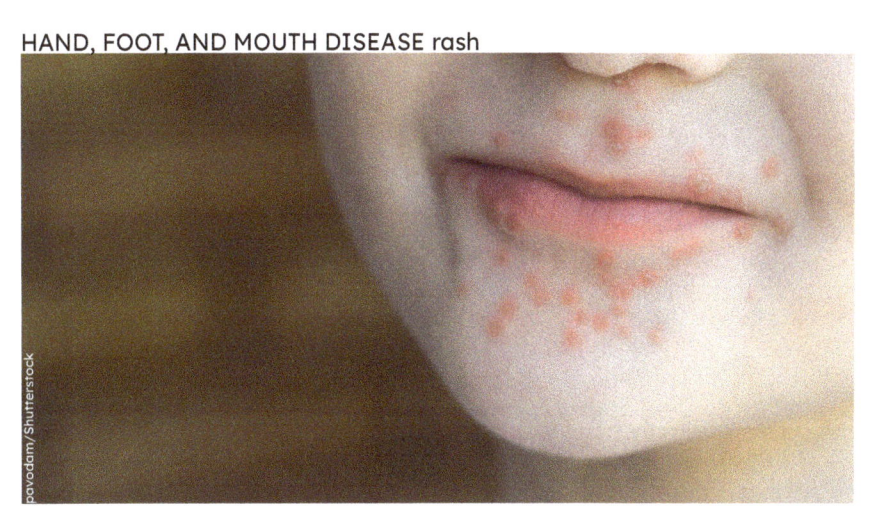

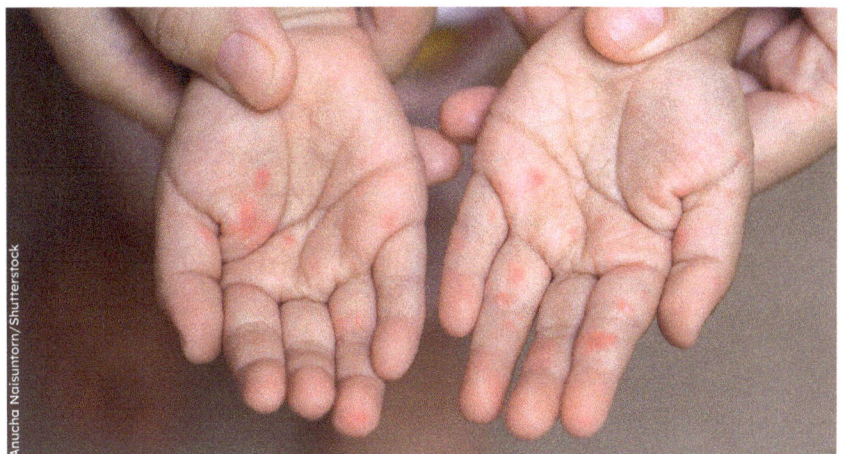

HAND, FOOT, AND MOUTH DISEASE rash

## SYMPTOMS:

- Fever may be present, but not in all cases.
- Nasal symptoms may be present.
- Blisters around the mouth, in the mouth and on the hands and feet develop one to two days after the initial symptoms. The rash can also be present on the buttocks to a significant extent in some cases.
- Mouth and throat pain may be present – and because of this, drooling may be present (the child does not want to swallow because of the pain).

## WHAT TO DO AT HOME:

- Treat the fever and pain with acetaminophen or ibuprofen as needed.
- Encourage fluid intake; your child may not want to drink because of the pain, so small frequent amounts may be helpful. Avoid giving any carbonated or citrus drinks – these will cause increased mouth and throat pain. Food such as yogurt, pudding, ice cream and jello may be comforting.
- There is no treatment for the blisters themselves; they will go away on their own.

## WHEN TO CONTACT YOUR CHILD'S HEALTHCARE PROVIDER

- **If you are unsure of the diagnosis.**
- **If your child has had a known exposure and is experiencing the symptoms mentioned above, you may choose not to contact your child's healthcare provider if you feel confident in managing the illness at home.**

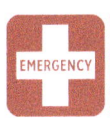

## WHEN TO GO TO THE EMERGENCY ROOM

- **Normally, it would not be necessary to be seen in the Emergency Room with this condition.**
- **Contact your child's provider first to get recommendations.**

## DIAGNOSIS AND TREATMENT:

- A physical examination by your child's provider will be able to confirm the diagnosis. No additional testing will be necessary. There is not a specific treatment for this condition; acetaminophen or ibuprofen can be used for the fever and discomfort that comes with this condition.

## IMPORTANT:

- A person is contagious from the time the illness starts until the blisters have all popped and are drying.
- This virus infection is spread by mouth and nasal secretions; washing hands helps decrease the spread. The virus is also shed in a child's stools – so extra care should be taken when changing dirty diapers.
- This is usually an infection in infants and toddlers; however, older children and adults can have it too.
- A child may return to school, daycare or babysitter's when fever has been been gone for 24-48 hours and all lesions are in a "drying-up" stage.

# IMPETIGO:

- Very common in children.
- Typically occurs during warmer months of the year.
- Easily transmitted from one place to another, either on the person who has it or to someone else; spread is by direct contact with the sore.

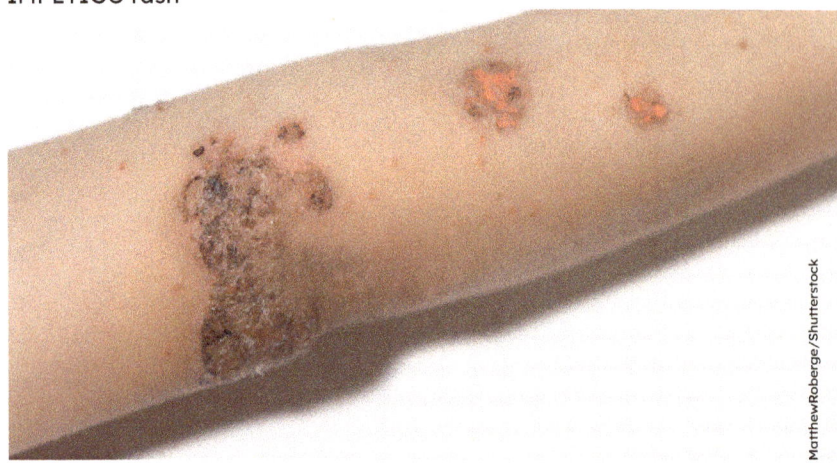

IMPETIGO rash

## CAUSES:

- Impetigo is a bacterial infection in the top layers of the skin, usually caused by either a Strep or Staph bacteria.

## SYMPTOMS:

- Appears as either blisters or sores initially; can ooze a liquid material and then form either a "crusted honey" top or a thicker wet looking crust. Sores can be found anywhere on the body.
- The nose can be a source of impetigo in children; there will be sores seen at the opening of the nostrils and often spreading outward on the face.

## WHAT TO DO AT HOME:

- Clean daily the areas with anti-bacterial soap carefully so as not to spread the infection.
- Keep any sore that is actively draining covered with a bandaid to prevent spread of infection.
- To prevent spread to others, wash any towels, wash rags, bedding and clothes that have been in contact with the sores.

## DIAGNOSIS AND TREATMENT:

- Your child's medical provider can usually make the diagnosis by visual inspection.
- If there are just a few spots, they can usually be successfully treated with a topical antibiotic ointment; if there are numerous lesions, an oral antibiotic is usually needed.

## WHEN IS THE CHILD NO LONGER CONTAGIOUS:

- The child is no longer contagious 24 hours after antibiotic therapy has started and when there are no draining sores.

### WHEN TO CONTACT YOUR CHILD'S HEALTHCARE PROVIDER

- **When there are more than 3-4 spots that you feel are impetigo (treatment will need to be prescribed by the provider).**

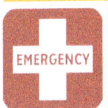

### WHEN TO GO TO THE EMERGENCY ROOM

- **Normally, it would not be necessary to be seen in the Emergency Room with this condition.**
- **Contact your child's provider first to get recommendations.**

# MOLLUSCUM CONTAGIOSUM:

> Molluscum Contagiosum is a viral infection that can affect individuals of all ages, but is commonly found in toddlers and children.

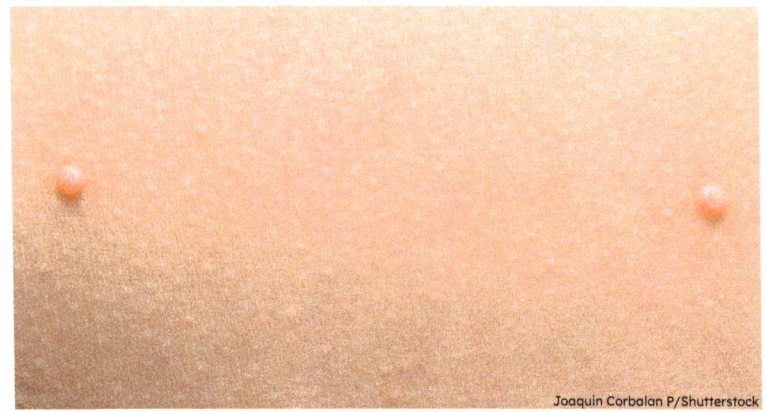

MOLLUSCUM CONTAGIOSUM rash

## CAUSE:

- The virus responsible for this infection is a Pox virus, similar to the Smallpox virus.

## SYMPTOMS:

- Lesions can appear on any part of the body except for the palms of the hands and the soles of the feet.
- Usually appear as single dome-shaped white or flesh-colored bumps. When the dome of the lesion is opened, a cheesy white material is released, which is the contagious component.
- Spread to other parts of the body can occur when the cheesy material is spread around the affected area or through hand contact with other body parts.
- The virus can also be transmitted to others who come in close contact with the cheesy material. Fortunately, there is no evidence that Molluscum C. can be transmitted in a swimming pool.
- A child may have just a few lesions or hundreds of lesions.

## WHAT TO DO AT HOME:

- There are no over-the-counter medications to treat Molluscum Contagiosum.
- Try to keep clothing over the warts so as to prevent transmission to others.
- Cover lesions in open areas with an adhesive bandage if possible.
- Try to prevent your child from scratching the lesions; opening the lesions will spread the infection and cause more lesions.

## WHEN TO CONTACT YOUR CHILD'S HEALTHCARE PROVIDER

- **If you are unsure if what your child has is Molluscum Contagiosum.**
- **If your child has many lesions and you are frustrated.**

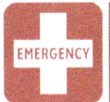

## WHEN TO GO TO THE EMERGENCY ROOM

- **Normally, it would not be necessary to be seen in the Emergency Room with this condition.**

## WHAT IS DONE TO EVALUATE/DIAGNOSE/TREAT THIS CONDITION:

- A physical examination by your child's provider can usually make the diagnosis.
- Treatment: involves topical therapy, such as acid or other destructive agent being applied directly to the bumps; this is done by a physician.
- Lesions can resolve on their own!! – anywhere from a few months up to a year.

## SCABIES:

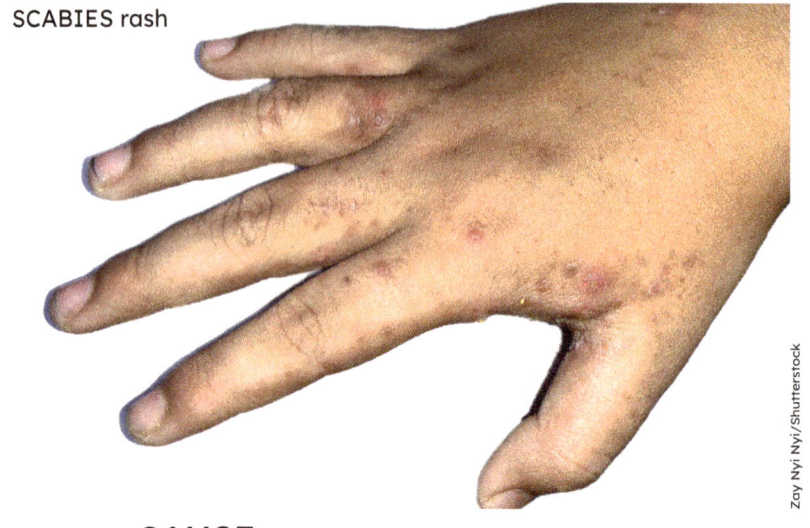

SCABIES rash

### CAUSE:

- A skin infestation caused by the mite Sarcoptic Scabiei.
- Incubation period (time from exposure to appearance of symptoms) can be 4-8 weeks.
- Scabies is spread through prolonged skin to skin contact with an infected person, or occasionally by sharing bedclothes, towels, or other items with a person who has Scabies. Trying on clothes at a clothing store has also been noted as a potential source of scabies.

### SYMPTOMS:

- Intense itching is present.
- Raised bumps, can be flush or pink colored.
- Tracts under the skin can sometimes be seen in between the bumps.
- Typically occurs on the trunk but can be found on the arms and legs. In infants, lesions may appear on the face and scalp as well.

## WHAT CAN BE DONE AT HOME:

- Can treat itching with antihistamines - Claritin® (loratadine), Zyrtec® (cetirizine), or Benadryl®. Itching may occur for several weeks after treatment with the prescription cream.
- Enviromental control – see below for in-depth recommendations.
- Treatment for scabies involves a prescription lotion or cream, which should be applied as directed by a physician.
- When Scabies is diagnosed, it is recommended that all family members be treated at the same time.

## WHEN TO CONTACT YOUR CHILD'S HEALTHCARE PROVIDER

- **When you suspect that the rash is scabies.**
- **When your child has an <u>extremely</u> itchy rash**

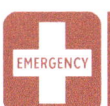

## WHEN TO GO TO THE EMERGENCY ROOM

- **Normally, it would not be necessary to be seen in the Emergency Room with this condition.**

## WHAT IS DONE TO EVALUATE/DIAGNOSE/TREAT THIS CONDITION:

- Your child's medical provider most often will be able to make the diagnosis after performing a physical examination of your child's skin.
- Occasionally, the diagnosis is not certain; a skin scraping of the rash can be sent to the lab, looking for the mite in the skin scraping.

- Treatment consists of applying permethrin 5% cream to the entire skin surface from neck down; it is left on for the recommended period of time – carefully read the directions that come with the cream. Permethrin cream is safe for anyone older than 2 months of age. (When treating infants and young children, the cream should be applied to the head and scalp as well). Permethrin has to be prescribed by a medical provider; there are no over-the-counter medications available.
- The itching from scabies is caused by a hypersensitivity reaction to the body and/or feces of the mite in the skin; occasionally a steroid cream or oral steroid are helpful with the management of the itching.
- After treatment, the patient should put on clean clothes, sleep on clean bedclothes, and use fresh towels.

## ENVIROMENTAL CONTROL:

- Clothing, bedding, and towels used by a person with scabies within the prior three days before treatment need to be washed in hot water and then dried on high heat in the dryer. Alternative options are dry cleaning these articles or sealing them in a plastic bag for 72 hours. It is felt that scabies mites cannot survive more than 2-3 days off human skin.
- Spraying insecticides on surfaces throughout the house is not indicated or recommended.

## EXTRA:

- It is important to mention that "mange" in dogs is caused by a different scabies mite; this mite can be transmitted to humans, but it cannot survive on humans.
Therefore, it cannot cause skin infections in humans.

# The Skin 167

# SHINGLES:

- More common than chicken pox in this era.

- Shingles can occur in anyone who has had chicken pox or who has had the chicken pox vaccine.

- Lesions or sores of shingles occur in an isolated area of the body ( could be one side of the face, one arm or one leg or one side of the trunk).

- Shingles occur along a major nerve serving a particular part of the body.

- Shingles look a little like chicken pox but the "spots" are usually in small groups and are smaller than chicken pox spots.

- Spots have a red base with tiny blisters on top.

- Shingles can sometimes be confused with poison ivy due to its appearance.

- A person can get shingles more than once.

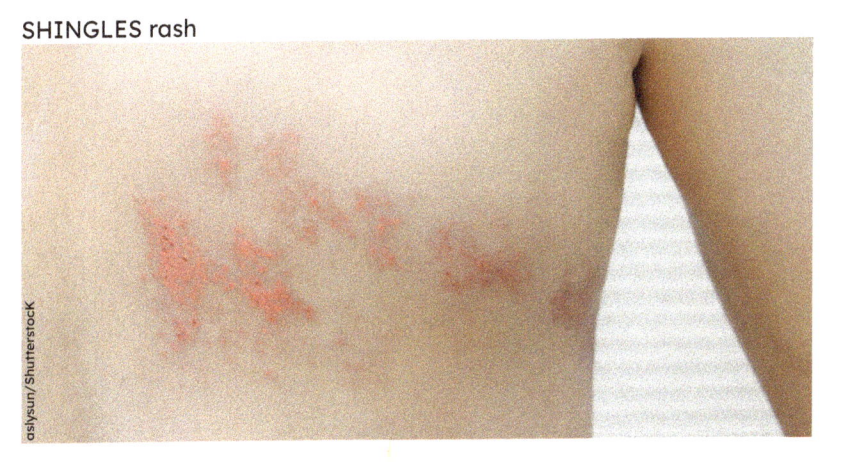

SHINGLES rash

## SYMPTOMS:

- Shingles do not normally cause any symptoms in a healthy child except for itching and maybe some tingling in the area.
- Shingles causing pain in children is uncommon, unlike in adults.
- It is uncommon for children to run a fever or feel ill with shingles.
- Shingles in adults can be very painful and prolonged, with pain lasting for months after an outbreak. Adults may also feel unwell with shingles, which differs from children.

## WHEN TO CONTACT YOUR CHILD'S HEALTHCARE PROVIDER

- **The rash of shingles can be confused with poison ivy, therefore the diagnosis of shingles needs to be made by a healtcare provider.**
- **If diagnosed within 48-72 hours of rash development, treatment may be given.**

## TREATMENT:

- If child is seen within 48-72 hours of breakout, an anti-viral medication can be prescribed. This will shorten the length of time that lesions are present as well as minimize itching and/or pain from shingles.
- Itching can be treated with an anti-itch medication like Benadryl® or long acting antihistamine.
- Prescription medications can be given in the case of pain associated with shingles.
- Lesions of shingles do not need to be directly treated.

## HOW LONG IS THE CHILD CONTAGIOUS:

- Once all lesions are scabbed, the child is no longer contagious.
- If the lesions can be covered with clothing until all are scabbed over (normally 7-10 days), the child does not need to isolate.
- If lesions are on the face, the child needs to isolate until all lesions are scabbed over.
- It is felt that a person is contagious 24 hours prior to the breakout of the lesions.
- A person with shingles can "cause" a chicken pox infection in a child who is not yet immunized against chicken pox or in one who is immune-compromised.

# 170 The Skin

## COMMON WARTS:

- Common warts are caused by the Human Papilloma Virus (HPV). The strains of HPV that cause common warts are not associated with cancer-producing strains of HPV.

- They typically appear as small, grainy bumps on the hands and feet, but they can occur elsewhere on the body as well. Warts on the bottom of the feet are referred to as "plantar warts".

- Common warts can be contagious if scratched or touched; they can spread to another part of the body.

- Children and young adults are more likely to develop common warts due to their lack of protective immunity to the HPV virus.

**COMMON WARTS**

# DIAGNOSIS AND TREATMENT:

- While most people prefer to treat warts for cosmetic reasons, treatment is not always necessary.
- However, if treatment is desired, it can be done through a variety of methods such as cryotherapy (freezing) or acid application (either with over the counter products or by a physician).
  Over the counter acid preparations come in both liquids and paste options.
  One applies the acid to the wart, covers it well with a water proof type tape and leaves it in place for 48 hours. Remove the tape and then wash the treated area. Allow for several days in between treatments. Using a disposable file (like an Emery board) file away the dead skin white area) on top of the wart and then reapply more acid preparation and repeat the process until the wart is gone.
- Typically, several rounds of treatment (up to a month's worth) are required to fully eradicate the wart.
- The above described treatment can be used on any type of common wart — both plantar warts and those anywhere else.
- Warts will typically resolve on their own over time without any treatment as well — one just has to be patient.

# RASHES THAT ARE FLAT:

## COMMON DIAPER RASH:

### CAUSES:

- Occurs in infants who are in diapers.
- These can be caused by being in a dirty diaper for too long, irritation and chafing of the diaper on baby's skin, starting solid foods, diarrhea, and breastfeeding (frequent stools).

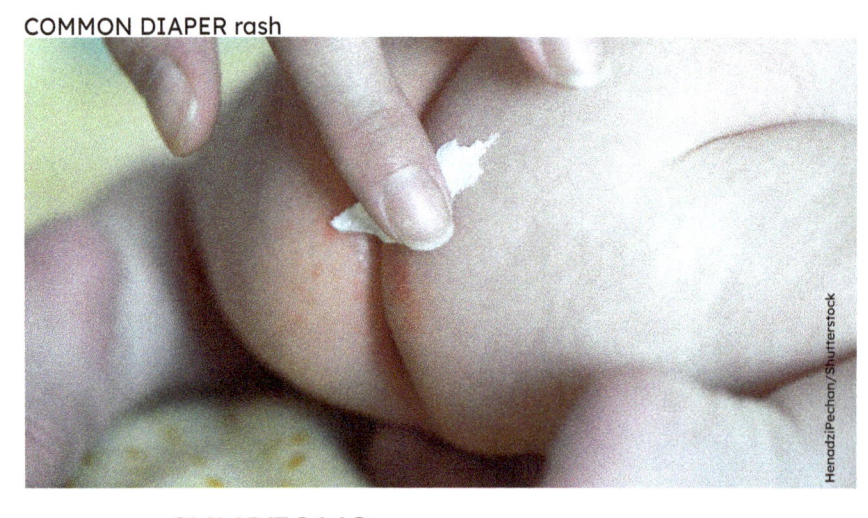

COMMON DIAPER rash

### SYMPTOMS:

- This rash usually is flat and red and does not get into into the skin folds — in contrast to a yeast diaper rash.
- The rash is present in areas where stool frequently comes in contact with the skin (on the inner buttocks on either side of the rectum) or in areas where the diaper is normally more wet from urine (in the front diaper area below the top of the diaper).
- This type of diaper rash can be very frustrating at times to clear; in addition, it frequently returns.

## WHAT TO DO AT HOME:

- Clean the area of rash with tap water - DO NOT USE BABY WIPES.
- Change the diaper often.
- If possible, let the area air dry for a while.
- Apply an over-the-counter diaper cream, ointment or petroleum jelly on the area involved.
Zinc oxide is a good skin barrier that can be used when the rash is very red and the skin looks raw. It does not have to be wiped off at diaper changes.

## WHEN TO CONTACT YOUR CHILD'S HEALTHCARE PROVIDER

- **When the diaper rash is not improving with your home treatment.**
- **If the rash starts bleeding.**
- **If your child is quite uncomfortable with the diaper rash.**

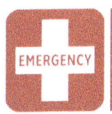

## WHEN TO GO TO THE EMERGENCY ROOM

- **Diaper rashes should not require an Emergency Room visit.**

## WHAT IS DONE TO EVALUATE/DIAGNOSE/TREAT THIS CONDITION:

- A description of the rash, a picture of the rash sent to the medical provider or a quick physical examination can quickly make the diagnosis.
- There are no prescription medications for this type of diaper rash. The prescription used for a yeast diaper rash does not help this type of diaper rash.
- The medical provider may be able to suggest some ideas that you have not yet tried.

# YEAST DIAPER RASH:

## CAUSES:

- A fungus infection of the skin, normally Candida.
- Can occur after the infant has been on an antibiotic
- Warm, moist areas are common locations for this rash to occur.

**YEAST DIAPER rash**

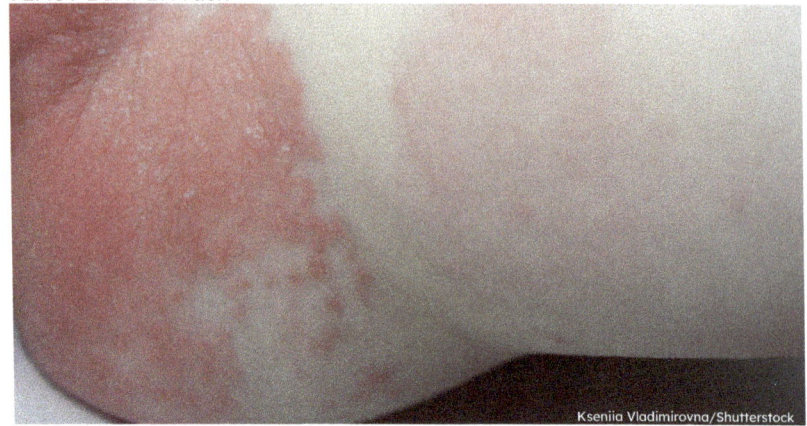

## SYMPTOMS:

- Yeast diaper rashes are usually seen in infants who are in diapers and less than one year of age; these rashes are rare after two yars of age.
- The rash is usually located in the diaper area in the skin folds, on the genitalia, and on the lower abdomen and very upper thighs.
- The rash consists of raised, bright red bumps that appear shiny that then come together to create a larger area. There are "satellite bumps" spreading out from the border of the main rash.

## WHAT TO DO AT HOME:

- An over-the-counter antifungal cream (clotrimazole or miconazole) can be tried first before contacting your child's medical provider.

## WHEN TO CONTACT YOUR CHILD'S HEALTHCARE PROVIDER

- **When the diaper rash is not improving with an over-the-counter antifungal medication.**

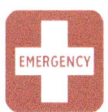

## WHEN TO GO TO THE EMERGENCY ROOM

- **Diaper rashes should not require an Emergency Room visit.**

## DIAGNOSIS AND TREATMENT:

- This rash is common in infants; either a description of where the rash is, a picture sent in to your child's provider's office, or a direct physical examination can easily help make the diagnosis.
- A prescription antifungal cream or ointment can be prescribed to treat this type of diaper rash.

# FIFTH DISEASE (ERYTHEMA INFECTIOSUM):

## CAUSE:

- The Parvovirus B19 is responsible for this infection. (NOTE: only humans can be infected with this specific virus type; dogs and cats can be infected with other parvoviruses, but these types do not infect humans). Fifth Disease usually occurs anytime from late winter to early summer. Every 3-4 years, there are outbreaks when significant numbers of children are affected. This virus normally infects toddlers and grade school aged children.

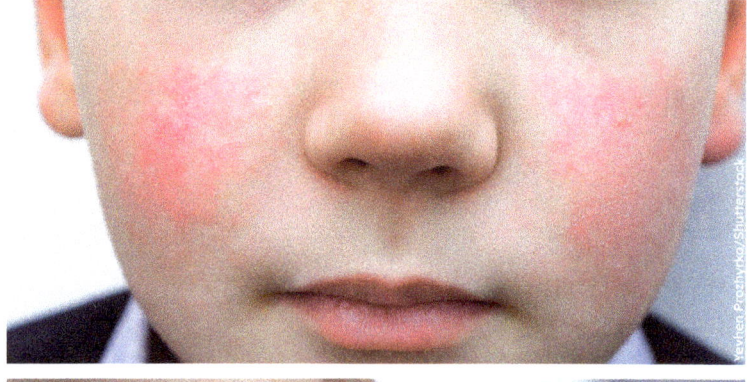

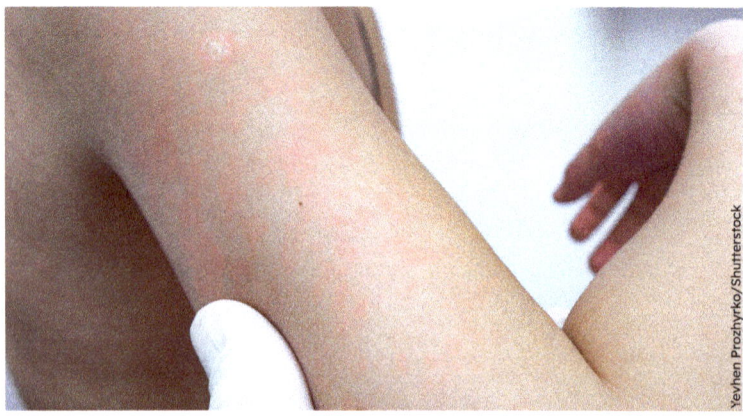

**FIFTH DISEASE rash**

## SYMPTOMS:

- During the time that the child is contagious with the virus, there are no symptoms.
- The classic rash appears after the actual virus infection; the first rash that appears is the "slapped cheeks" rash – a flat, bright red rash on both cheeks. It will blanch (disappears temporarily when pushed on).
- Within the next 1-2 days after the "slapped cheeks" rash, a pink-red rash develops on the trunk and extremities. This rash is referred to as "reticular' – it appears "lacy" (as if the child had laid out in the sun covered with a lace tablecloth).
- The rash may itch from time to time.

## WHAT TO DO AT HOME:

- There is no treatment for this rash.

### WHEN TO CONTACT YOUR CHILD'S HEALTHCARE PROVIDER

- **If you are unsure of the diagnosis, contact your child's provider. It is not necessary to have your child seen with this condition, unless there are other circumstances present.**

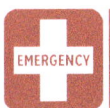

### WHEN TO GO TO THE EMERGENCY ROOM

- **This rash does not require an Emergency Room visit. If you have concerns, contact your child's healthcare provider first before going to the Emergency Room.**

## DIAGNOSIS AND TREATMENT:

- A physical examination by the provider will confirm the diagnosis; there is no additional testing necessary.

- There is no specific treatment that can be prescribed for this condition.

## EXTRA:

- A child is not contagious during this rash; there is no indication for staying home from school or daycare.
- Normally a child will develop immunity to this virus after the first episode, thus no subsequent infections should occur.
- If a pregnant woman is exposed to a child with Erythema Infectiosum, she needs to notify her obstetrician promptly. There is a slight increased risk of pregnancy complications associated with exposure to the Parvovirus B19 that causes Fifth disease.

# HIVES (URTICARIA)

- Also known as known as "welts"; can appear on the skin and vary in size from small patches to several inches in diameter.
- Can be smooth and slightly raised, either skin-colored or light pink.
- Can come and go in a matter of minutes to a few hours.
- Are usually quite itchy.

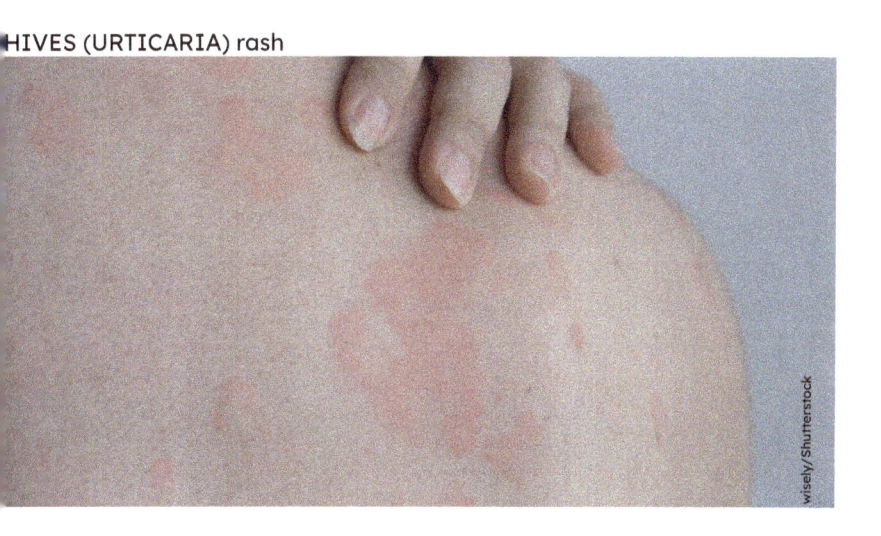

HIVES (URTICARIA) rash

## CAUSES:

- An allergic reaction to food, insect stings, or medication.
- A recent viral infection is the most common cause of hives in children. Following a viral infection, hives may persist for several days to several weeks.

## SYMPTOMS:

- Itchy.
- Shortness of breath, lip swelling, and wheezing may occur with hives. If hives are accompanied by these symptoms, seek medical attention immediately.
- Hives associated with a virus infection are not associated with any other symptoms.

## WHAT TO DO AT HOME:

- If hives are associated with shortness of breath, lip swelling and/or wheezing, give a dose of Benadryl® as soon as possible (see dosage chart in Appendix).
- If hives are not associated with any other symptoms, antihistamines such as Benadryl®, cetirizine, or loratadine (see dosage chart in Appendix) may be used as treatment for the hives and itching. If no improvement is seen after several days, call your child's medical provider. Additional medications may be added.

## IMPORTANT:

- ***** *Steroids are not indicated in viral caused hives******

### WHEN TO CONTACT YOUR CHILD'S HEALTHCARE PROVIDER

- **When hives are still present 3-5 days after starting Benadryl®, cetirizine, or loratadine.**

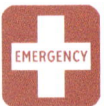

### WHEN TO GO TO THE EMERGENCY ROOM

- **When there are symptoms of shortness of breath, wheezing, lip swelling, and/or vomiting.**

# MEASLES AND RUBELLA (GERMAN MEASLES):

## CAUSES:
- Measles is caused by the Morbillivirus.
- Rubella is caused by the Rubella virus.
- Both illnesses are very uncommon today.

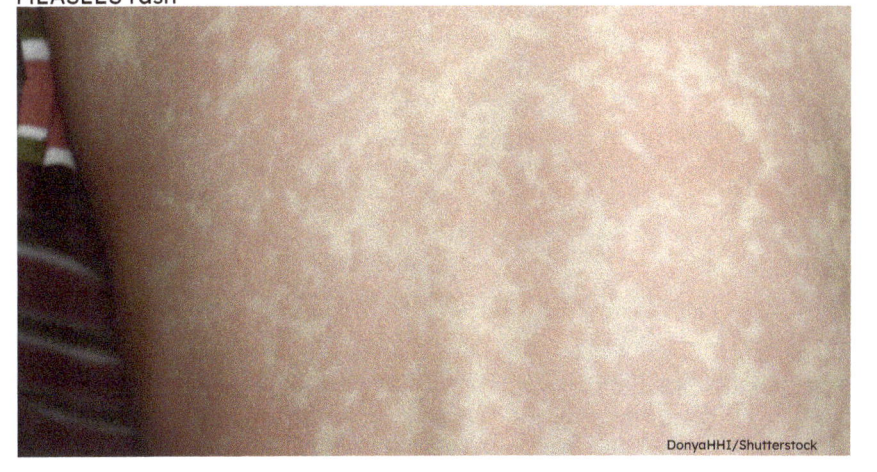

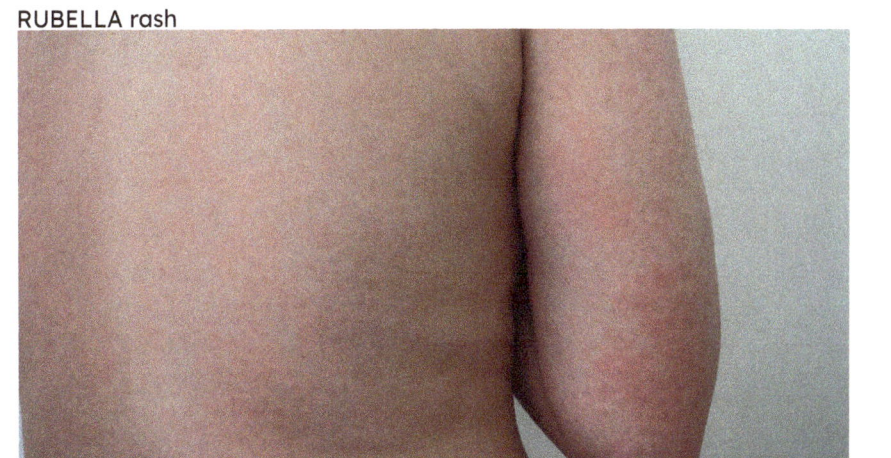

MEASLES rash

RUBELLA rash

## SYMPTOMS:

- Measle symptoms include high fever, cough, conjunctivitis (red eyes), runny nose, and a blotchy red rash (all at the same time). The rash normally starts 3 -5 days after the other symptoms have started; the fever can get quite high (104 degrees) when the rash starts.
  The main symptoms last about 7 days.
- Measles rash starts as flat red spots on the face and around the ears, then spreads to the rest of the body; the rash does not itch.
- Rubella symptoms include mild fever, cough, runny nose, sore throat, tender lymph nodes in the back of the neck and ears, and rash.
  The main symptoms last about 3 days.
- The rash of Rubella starts as a light pink spotty rash on the face, and then spreads to the trunk and extremities.

## WHAT TO DO AT HOME:

- Treat the symptoms, particularly the fever.
- Insure your child is taking in adequate fluids.
- As long as there is fever, your child needs to be isolated at home.
- IF YOU SUSPECT THAT YOUR CHILD MAY HAVE MEASLES OR RUBELLA (THE LIKELIHOOD IS VERY SLIM UNLESS YOUR CHILD IS UNVACCINATED) CALL YOUR CHILD'S MEDICAL PROVIDER.

### WHEN TO CONTACT YOUR CHILD'S HEALTHCARE PROVIDER

- **If you suspect that your child may have measles or rubella, contact your child's provider.**
- **Both are reportable conditions, therefore tests need to be done to confirm the diagnosis.**

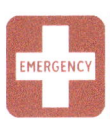

# WHEN TO GO TO THE EMERGENCY ROOM

- **Normally, it would not be necessary to be seen in the Emergency Room with this condition. Contact your child's healthcare provider first to get recommendations.**

## DIAGNOSIS AND TREATMENT:

- Your child's medical provider will take a history and perform a physical examination.
- If measles or rubella is suspected, a blood test will be needed to confirm the diagnosis.
- There is not a prescription medication for the treatment of measles and rubella.

## IMPORTANT:

- Both measles and rubella are preventable diseases; there are vaccines against both. The measles vaccine was introduced in 1963; the rubella vaccine was introduced in 1969. The combined mumps-measles-rubella vaccine became available in 1971. The vaccines are very effective; only individuals who have not been vaccinated against measles and rubella can contract these infections.
- Keep in mind that fever and rash are present together in measles and rubella; this contrasts with other viral caused rashes.
- Measles and rubella are contagious via the respiratory droplets of the patient; one needs to isolate until after all fever has resolved with both infections.

# PETECHIAE/PURPURA:

## CAUSES:

- A low platelet count (the blood cells that help with clotting) or a blood clotting defect problem.
- Certain medical conditions that cause "leaky" blood vessels.
- Increased pressure in blood vessels – some examples of this are pushing hard to deliver a baby, pushing hard to pass a hard bowel movement, having something wrapped too tight around an extremity.
- Trauma to an area.

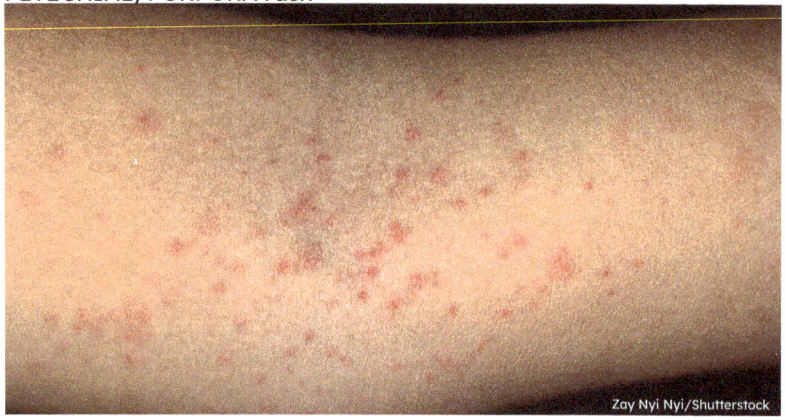

PETECHIAE/PURPURA rash

## SYMPTOMS:

- Petechiae are tiny "blood spots" either localized to an area or generalized over the body.
  They can change in color from red to purple-brown as they fade.
- Purpura are larger purplish spots (1/4 inch or bigger) either localized or generalized.
- If one pushes on either of these spots, they will not blanch (temporarily disappear); this is in contrast to most rashes that children experience.
- Neither petechiae nor purpura itch or hurt.

## WHAT TO DO AT HOME:

- Evaluate the location of these spots; it will help you decide if there is a need to call your child's medical provider.
- Lots of coughing, episodes of vomiting, pushing hard to have a bowel movement – these activities can cause petechiae to appear on the face, neck and upper chest.
- If your child had a tourniquet on for blood drawing purposes, the arm past the tourniquet could develop petechiae.
- Trauma to an area (getting hit, falling down) can cause petechiae or purpura to appear just in that area.
- The above situations are all appropriate. explanations of petechiae and purpura; you do not necessarily need to call your child's medical provider.

## DIAGNOSIS AND TREATMENT:

- The medical provider will take a history and perform a physical examination.
- Additional laboratory testing may be performed.
- Treatment plan and further recommendations will be dependent on the results of the provider's evaluation and laboratory studies.

## WHEN TO CONTACT YOUR CHILD'S HEALTHCARE PROVIDER

- If petechiae or purpura are generalized (extremities, trunk and face), contact your child's healthcare provider.
- If there are petechiae or purpura in locations for which you cannot readily explain, contact your child's healthcare provider.

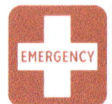

## WHEN TO GO TO THE EMERGENCY ROOM

- If you are directed to the Emergency Room by your child's medical provider.
- If you are concerned and you cannot contact your child's medical provider.
- If your child is not feeling well and/or has a fever with petechiae or purpura, call your child's provider or go to the Emergency Room.

# PITYRIASIS ROSEA:

## CAUSE:
- Unknown but thought to be a response to a virus infection.

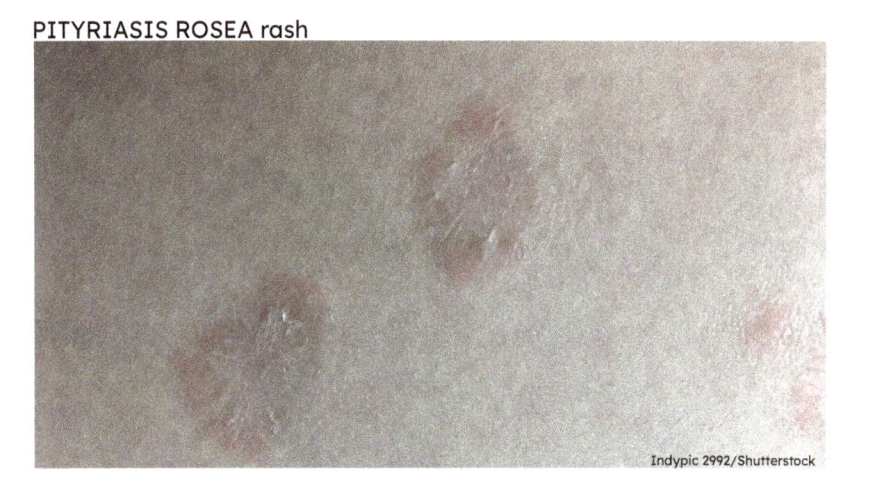

PITYRIASIS ROSEA rash

Indypic 2992/Shutterstock

## SYMPTOMS:
- The rash is itchy at times, especially after bathing or when a person is sweaty.
- It starts with a "herald patch" a circular to oval slightly raised pink lesion that is at least 1 inch in size and is found on the face, neck, or trunk.
- Within days, the remaining rash appears as slightly oval shaped, pinkish lesions that are minimally raised. They are scattered on the trunk primarily and are arranged in a fern-like or Christmas tree pattern. The rash can be found on the arms at times, as well as the face in some children.
- Depending on skin color, the lesions can be brown, purple, or gray in addition to pink.
- Typically, Pityriasis Rosea does not occur in children until after the 8th birthday.

## WHAT TO DO AT HOME:

- Treatment of the itching with Benadryl® or a long-acting antihistamine is recommended.

### WHEN TO CONTACT YOUR CHILD'S HEALTHCARE PROVIDER

- **When you are unsure of the diagnosis of the rash.**

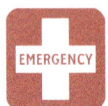

### WHEN TO GO TO THE EMERGENCY ROOM

- **Going to the Emergency Room for this rash is not necessary.**

## WHAT IS DONE TO EVALUATE/DIAGNOSE/TREAT THIS CONDITION:

- A physical examination performed by your child's medical provider can usually make the diagnosis.
- There is no testing that can or should be done.
- There is not a specific treatment for this rash; it will resolve over the course of several weeks.
- There are no recommendations for isolation while the rash is present.

# ROSEOLA:

> Normally seen in infants and toddlers.

## CAUSE:

- Human herpes virus 6 causes roseola.

ROSEOLA rash

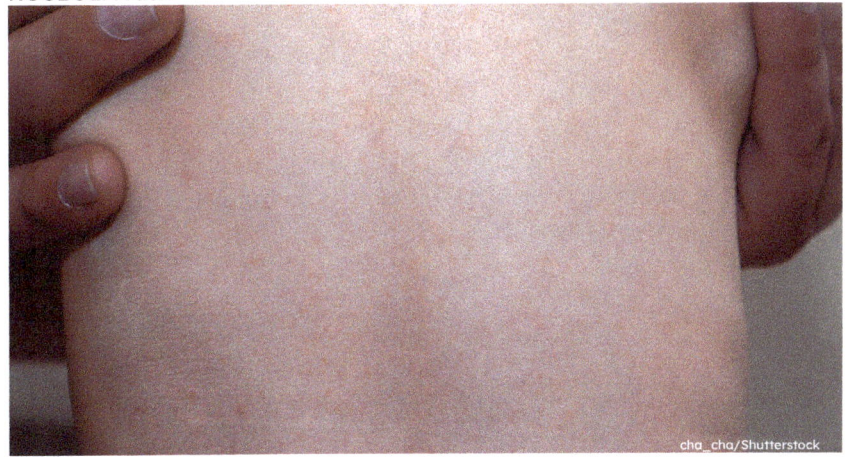

## SYMPTOMS:

- High fever for approximately 3 days (72 hours) occurs first.
- The child acts like he/she does not feel well.
- Typically, there are no other associated symptoms.
- Appetite and activity level may be decreased.
- 12 – 24 hours after the fever stops, the rash of roseola appears. The rash is a flat pink spotty rash that starts on the neck, and then spreads to the trunk and extremities. It is usually not itchy. The rash goes away in 3 days.

## WHAT TO DO AT HOME:

- Treat the fever as needed with acetaminophen or ibuprofen.
- Insure your child is taking in adequate fluids.
- As long as fever is present, your child needs to be isolated at home.
- There is no needed treatment for the rash.

## WHEN TO CONTACT YOUR CHILD'S HEALTHCARE PROVIDER

- **If fever persists for longer than 48-72 hours.**
- **If your child is not drinking adequately, is sleeping more than usual, or is having difficulty staying awake.**

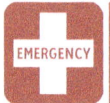

## WHEN TO GO TO THE EMERGENCY ROOM

- **If you are directed to the Emergency Room by your child's healthcare provider.**
- **If any of the above concerns are present and you cannot contact your child's healthcare provider.**

## DIAGNOSIS AND TREATMENT:

- A history and physical examination will be performed by the medical provider; depending on findings from this evaluation the provider may order laboratory testing to further evaluate.
- If the fever has resolved and the rash is present at the time of the provider visit, the diagnosis is easily made.
- There are no prescription medications indicated for roseola.

# SCARLET FEVER RASH:

## CAUSE:
- Certain strains of the Strep bacteria that cause strep throat and impetigo cause this rash.

## SYMPTOMS:
- This rash starts out as flat red blotches that spread and then develop a "sand paper" feel.
- The rash usually is present on the face (but sparing the area around the mouth), the neck, under the arms, and the trunk. The groin (or underpant area) can be fairly red as well.
- The rash can be itchy.
- It resolves spontaneously over several days. Occasionally a week after the rash one can see some peeling or flaking of the skin involved with the rash. This is normal.

## WHEN TO CONTACT YOUR CHILD'S HEALTHCARE PROVIDER
- **If you have any concerns about the rash.**
- **The rash of scarlet fever looks very different from a medication caused rash; any concerns that you have about a medication caused rash should be discussed with your child's medical provider.**

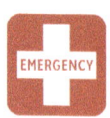

## WHEN TO GO TO THE EMERGENCY ROOM

- **This skin rash should not require a visit to the Emergency Room.**

## DIAGNOSIS AND TREATMENT:

- A description of the rash, a picture of the rash sent to your child's medical provider, or a physical examination will quickly provide the diagnosis.
- As above, no specific treatment is needed; make sure that your child completes the entire prescription of antibiotic for the strep infection.
- Once the child has been on antibiotic for the strep infection for 24 hours, isolation is not needed – even if the scarlet fever rash is present.

Scarlet fever (which is known for a characteristic rash) for many centuries was considered a deadly infection. In the 1920'ss it was discovered that scarlet fever was related to streptococcal infections (strep throat in particular); the rash of scarlet fever was caused by a toxin released by certain strains of strep bacteria.
Thus, prior to the development of antibiotics, people died from streptococcal infections, not from scarlet fever. So scarlet fever was misunderstood for many centuries. Today, we know it as just a rash that a person can sometimes have in association with a strep infection. And, fortunately, penicillin was discovered in the late 1920's which led to successful treatment of streptococcal infections and a drastic decline in the death rate due to such infections.

# VIRAL RASHES (non specified):

## CAUSES:
- Viruses other than those listed above.
There are many non-serious viruses that commonly cause "viral" rashes in children. At this point in time, there is not a readily available test to determine which virus is the cause.

## SYMPTOMS:
- The rash may be itchy.
- This type of rash <u>follows</u> a fever (if there is one); fever is not present at the time of the rash.
- The rash is pink-red and splotchy, flat and barely raised. It temporarily disappears if you push on it.
- The rash usually appears first around the neck and then moves down the trunk, usually fading below the waist. Will sometimes be seen on the arms and legs.
- The rash usually lasts just a few days but can sometimes last several weeks.
- It will sometimes be seen after a minor illness.

## WHAT TO DO AT HOME:
- Benadryl®, Claritin® or Zyrtec® are helpful for the itching.
- The rash does not need any particular treatment; it resolves on its own.

## WHEN TO CONTACT YOUR CHILD'S HEALTHCARE PROVIDER

‣ When you have concerns about the rash that your child has, and you are not confident that it is a viral rash.

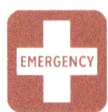

## WHEN TO GO TO THE EMERGENCY ROOM

‣ This skin condition should never require a visit to the Emergency Room.

## DIAGNOSIS AND TREATMENT:

‣ A physical examination by your child's provider should confirm the diagnosis; no testing is necessary.
‣ Treatment is primarily aimed at treating any itching that may be present.
‣ Your child is not contagious with this rash; school or daycare attendance is appropriate.

# RASHES THAT ARE SCALY/FLAKY:

## ECZEMA (ATOPIC DERMATITIS):

### CAUSES:
- Not known for sure.
- Multiple factors may play a role – the environment, genetic factors, and/or an "over active" immune system.

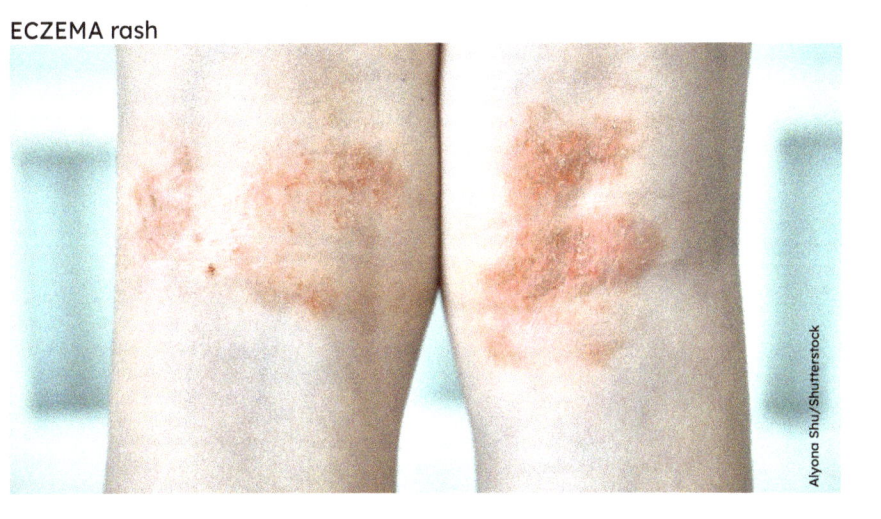

ECZEMA rash

### SYMPTOMS:
- Significant itching is present.
- Pink-red, dry patches may occur anywhere on the body.
- Patches may get scaly.
- Patches will sometimes crack from the dryness, weep fluid, and become crusty.
- The skin can sometimes become thickened.

## WHAT TO DO AT HOME:

- Make every attempt to keep your child's skin well hydrated with skin moisturizers on a daily basis. petroleum jelly is very helpful in extra dry areas.
- Follow the directions for medications that your child's provider or dermatologist prescribes. Keeping your child's skin moist and limiting scratching are very important. Consistent treatment is key to the success of managing eczema.
- Treat itching aggressively with Claritin®, Zyrtec® or Benadryl®.

## WHEN TO CONTACT YOUR CHILD'S HEALTHCARE PROVIDER

- **If your child has skin findings as described above and they are not improving with the care you are giving, contact your child's medical provider.**
- **When your child's eczema is worsening despite treating with prescription medication contact your child's healthcare provider.**

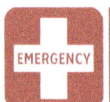

## WHEN TO GO TO THE EMERGENCY ROOM

- **This skin condition should never require a visit to the Emergency Room; if you have concerns, contact your child's provider first.**

## DIAGNOSIS AND TREATMENT:

- A physical examination by your child's provider should help clarify the diagnosis. Rarely are skin biopsies necessary.
- In addition to excellent skin care with daily moisturizers, steroid creams and ointments are recommended and prescribed by medical providers. For the majority of children with eczema, this will be sufficient care.
- When children do not improve with prescribed steroid creams and ointments, more intense treatment with immunosuppressants and biologic injectables are offered. Dermatologists are involved with a child's care at this point.

## EXTRAS:

- Eczema is not contagious; it cannot be spread from one person to another.
- Eczema is often associated with asthma and allergic rhinitis (hay fever) – "the allergy triad".
- Eczema does not have a cure at this point in time; however, as some children grow older, their eczema becomes much less active.

# RINGWORM:

## CAUSES:

- A superficial skin infection caused by several fungi - Trichophyton, Microsporum, or Epidermophyton.
- Sources of the fungi: soil, contaminated animals (young kittens in particular), infected humans.
- The name comes from a description of what the rash looks like - a "worm under the skin shaped like a ring", but, to clarify, the rash has nothing to do with worms.

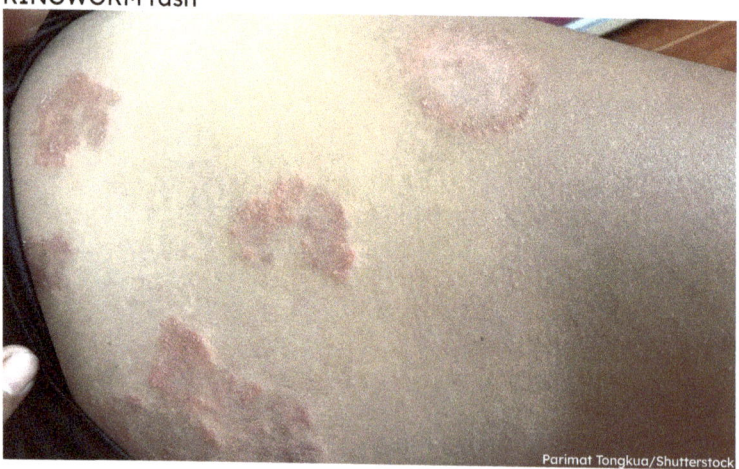

RINGWORM rash

## SYMPTOMS:

- An itchy, circular rash that has a more clear but scaly center with a raised red outer border; the rash can expand in size over time.

## WHAT TO DO AT HOME:

- If you suspect ringworm, you may try applying an over-the-counter cream (clotrimazole or miconazole) twice daily for one week; if there is no improvement, contact your child's healthcare provider.

## WHEN TO CONTACT YOUR CHILD'S HEALTHCARE PROVIDER

- If there has not been response to the over-the-counter treatment.
- If the rash is expanding in size or other spots are developing as well.

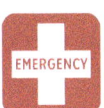

## WHEN TO GO TO THE EMERGENCY ROOM

- This skin condition should never require a visit to the Emergency Room.

## DIAGNOSIS AND TREATMENT:

- A physical examination performed by your child's medical provider usually clarifies the diagnosis. Occasionally a scraping of the rash is obtained and sent to the laboratory for confirmation.
- Treatment is a prescribed anti-fungal cream from a medical provider, particularly if an over-the-counter medication has already been tried.
- The rash remains contagious until 48 hours (about 2 days) after treatment is started; make every effort to keep it covered for that amount of time.
- Fungal infections of the skin can take upwards of at least one week after medication has started to improve and resolve.
- The same fungi that cause ringworm can also cause fungal infections in nails and on the scalp; these are more difficult to treat and usually require oral anti-fungal medication.
  If a fungal nail infection is suspected, a clipping of the nail is sent to the laboratory for confirmation before oral treatment is started.

# BURNS

## CAUSES:
- The sun, a hot object, fire, a chemical (certain cleaning products), and electricity are all causes of burns.

## DEGREE OF A BURN:
### (Dependent on how deep into the skin the injury is)
- <u>FIRST</u>: Only the very top layer of skin is affected. There is only redness of the burn area.
- <u>SECOND</u>: Involves the top layer of skin as well as part of the next layer of skin down. There is redness as well as a blister.
- <u>THIRD</u>: Involves the top layer of skin as well as the entire part of the next layer down. There is obvious loss of skin in the involved area.

## WHAT TO DO AT HOME:
FOR <u>FIRST</u> AND <u>SECOND</u> DEGREE BURNS:
- As soon as possible after the injury, run cold water over the involved area for 15 minutes.
- Give acetaminophen or ibuprofen for pain.
- Apply a topical burn relief spray or gel that contains lidocaine (avoid putting this on open wounds) as directed on the product.
- If there is open skin, apply some antibiotic ointment and cover it with gauze.
- Clean the affected area daily with an antibacterial soap and reapply antibiotic ointment to any open skin. Keep it covered until it looks healed.
  **Never clean burns with peroxide.**

- First and second degree burns normally heal in 7-10 days.
- The affected skin will flake or peel as part of the healing process.

FOR THIRD DEGREE BURNS:
- Do not attempt to clean or treat these burns at home.
- **If possible, cover the area with a clean wet cloth.**

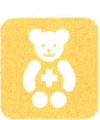

## WHEN TO CONTACT YOUR CHILD'S HEALTHCARE PROVIDER

- **When a second-degree burn is the size of the child's palm or larger.**
- **When a second-degree burn is present on the face, the external genitalia, the buttocks, or over a joint.**

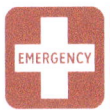

## WHEN TO GO TO THE EMERGENCY ROOM

- **Your child has a third-degree burn.**
- **Your child has extensive second degree burns.**
- **Your child has an electrical burn. Even though the burn may not be very large or a third degree burn, the child needs to be assessed for damage to internal organs caused by the electrical current.**

# PREVENTION OF BURNS:

- **SUN BURNS:**

    - **Sunscreen** is approved for all children older than 6 months of age; to prevent sunburn, it is important to apply sunscreen to your child (ren) whenever they are outside for more than just a few minutes in the sun. This includes all activities – swimming, sports, routine play. NOTE: being at a higher elevation than sea level increases the risk of sunburn).

## The Skin

- **SPF 50** is the recommended sunscreen rating for children.
- Sunscreen clothing is an acceptable alternative to sunscreen; remember to still apply sunscreen to open skin.
- Sun hats are also recommended for infants and toddlers to protect their scalps.
- Remember to reapply sunscreen every few hours – especially if your child is swimming or is sweating.

### BURNS FROM HOT OBJECTS/FIRES:

- Any objects that get hot that children like to grab (curling irons for example) need to be turned off and unplugged when not in use. Being put out of reach of children lessens the danger as well.
- Metal playground equipment (slides, for example) can get very hot on warm, sunny days. Make sure to check out the equipment before allowing your child to play on it.
- Do not allow your young children to be around your stove and oven when using the appliances for cooking and baking.
- Hot water from a faucet can be dangerous as well. Make sure that your water heater is set at 120 degrees F.
- Avoid having hot liquids sitting on tables and counters where toddlers can reach them and pull them over – spilling the hot liquid down the front of the body.
- When grilling outdoors, keep all children away from the hot grill.
- Keep all matches and lighters hidden from children.

### ELECTRICAL BURNS:

- Electrical burns occur when children (toddlers) bite into electrical cords or stick metal objects into electrical outlets – make sure that all electrical outlets have safety covers and attempt to keep all electrical cords hidden.

# SCRAPES AND CUTS

## CAUSES:
- Children being active.

## WHAT TO DO AT HOME:
- Clean the wound gently but well with antibacterial soap.
- **Do not use peroxide to clean open wounds; it is felt that peroxide can damage tissue.**
- **Do not use alcohol to clean wounds.**
- Apply an antibiotic ointment to the area and keep it covered until it has healed or has scabbed over.
- Make sure to clean the wound daily. Soaking in the bathtub is a helpful way to clean wounds.
- For superficial cuts, apply a band aid perpendicular to the cut. This will provide traction, keeping the edges of the cut together.

### WHEN TO CONTACT YOUR CHILD'S HEALTHCARE PROVIDER
- **When the cut is longer than ½ inch and/or fairly deep.**

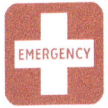

### WHEN TO GO TO THE EMERGENCY ROOM
- **When there is a cut greater than 1 inch in length and or deep.**
- **When the cut will not stop bleeding after 10 minutes of firm pressure.**

# ANIMAL BITES

## CAUSES:

- Dog bites and cat bites are the most common animal bites.
- If you live in a more rural area, skunks and raccoons are other animals that can inflict bites.
- Animal bites typically occur on the hands or the face in children.

## WHAT TO DO AT HOME:

- Wash the involved areas of skin very well with anti-bacterial soap and water.
- Flushing the area with lots of water is important.
- For scratches, apply an anti-bacterial ointment to them twice daily until they are healed.
- If the injury is only scratches, care can be rendered at home.

### WHEN TO CALL YOUR CHILD'S PROVIDER OR GO TO THE EMERGENCY ROOM IF THE PROVIDER IS NOT AVAILABLE

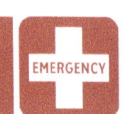

- **If there are skin punctures or cuts as a result of the animal bite, contact your child's provider or go to the Emergency Room within 12 hours after the injury. Both dog and cat bites have a high risk of becoming infected, so it will be important that an antibiotic be started.**
- **If there are animal bites on the face, these require the evaluation of a plastic surgeon; your child's provider or the Emergency Room should make the referral.**
- **MAKE SURE TO COMPLETE THE ANTIBIOTIC PRESCRIPTION GIVEN FOR YOUR CHILD'S ANIMAL BITE.**

# The Skin

## IMPORTANT NOTES:

- Dog bites in many municipalities require a report to the local police department – particularly if the dog that bit your child is not known to your family. This will expedite finding out the rabies immunization status of the dog.
- Your child may need a booster of the tetanus vaccine if it has been a certain amount of time since the last booster; your child's provider will make that determination.
- If your child has been bitten by an animal that lives in the "wild" (a skunk, a raccoon, a bat, or other similar animal), it is very important that your local county Health Department be notified; a risk assessment for potential rabies exposure will need to be done. If your child (or anyone else you know) is bitten by a bat, it is very important to catch the bat so that it can be assessed for rabies.

# MOSQUITO BITES

## CAUSE:

- Late spring, all summer, and early fall for most parts of the country is prime time for the mosquito to be the pest it is — causing many bites.

## WHAT TO DO AT HOME:

- Apply a cold pack to the area that has been bitten; this can help reduce the reaction to the mosquito bite.
- For itching, give your child either a short acting antihistamine (Benadryl®) or long acting antihistamine (cetirizine, loratadine) as directed
- Apply a topical hydrocortisone 1% cream (which is over the counter) to the bite/s twice daily; this can be quite helpful for minimizing the itching.
- Reactions to mosquito bites can be fairly intense at times – with **local** warmth, pinkness and swelling. Fortunately, mosquito bites will not cause a generalized allergic reaction with shortness of breath, lip swelling, or more serious complications.
- Your child's medical provider may prescribe a prescription strength steroid cream to help further if the 1% hydrocortisone cream is not relieving the symptoms.

## IMPORTANT NOTE:

- **Prevention** is the best way to avoid mosquito bites; child -approved insect sprays or lotions applied to the child's skin is quite helpful for prevention. The most important ingredient of these products is DEET (at a 30% concentration or less). Having your child wear long sleeves and pants when outside in the evening is very helpful as well.

# TICK BITES

## CAUSES:

- Depending on where you live in the United States, there are a variety of ticks that are present in the outdoors (usually found in tall grasses, weeds, and woods). All ticks are capable of carrying organisms (bacteria, viruses, and parasites) that they can then transmit to humans during a bite.
- There are two ways that someone may acquire a tick (or ticks) – either directly from the outdoors or indirectly from exposure to a family pet who goes outside.

## IMPORTANT FACT:

- A tick will come in contact with human skin either directly or indirectly via the persons' clothing or hair. Once on the skin, the tick will crawl around and ultimately bite the human and become attached. This normally does not happen immediately, but usually several hours after initial contact. The tick will feed on the human and eventually may inject fluids into the skin. It is the fluid that contains bacteria, viruses or parasites.

## WHAT TO DO AT HOME:

- Inspect your child's skin after playing outside on a daily basis (if you live in an area where ticks are found}. Make sure to inspect the scalp, ears, belly button, and all remaining skin – ticks will migrate **anywhere**. If you find one, remove it. Do not be afraid to touch the tick – grab its body (with either your fingers or tweezers) and pull it up and off. The entire body is normally removed – it may pull a tiny piece of skin with it. Make sure to dispose of the tick – but do not squeeze it prior to doing so. If by chance the tick's head is left in the skin as you pull a tick off, the chance of tick-borne disease is **not increased**. Rather, a minor local skin infection or reaction may occur. Clean the bite area with anti-bacterial soap and water after tick removal.

- After you have removed a tick, observe your child over the next several days for fever, headache, muscle aches, a spotty red rash on the legs or a bullseye lesion. If any of these symptoms do develop, call your child's provider immediately.
- Occasionally the area where the tick was removed can develop a slightly raised pink bump that may be itchy. This is just a local reaction - not an indication of infection from the tick. This does not require treatment.

## WHEN TO CONTACT YOUR CHILD'S HEALTHCARE PROVIDER URGENTLY

- **If any of the following symptoms occur in your child up to one week after removing a tick:**
  - Fever.
  - Headache.
  - Muscle aches.
  - Red/purple spotty rash.
  - A bullseye lesion at the tick bite site (this may take up to 30 days to appear after a tick bite).

**Make sure to mention to the child's healthcare provider that there was a tick exposure.**

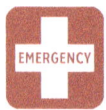

## WHEN TO GO TO THE EMERGENCY ROOM

- **If the above symptoms are present and you are not able to contact your child's provider, go to the Emergency Room. Make sure to mention to the E.R. staff that there was a tick exposure.**

## DIAGNOSIS AND TREATMENT:

- Your child's medical provider will perform a physical examination after taking a detailed history. An important piece of history is the geographic location where the tick bite occurred, as ticks carry different diseases in different geographical areas of the United States.
- If a tick-borne infection is suspected, blood tests can be performed to help confirm the diagnosis.
- If a tick-borne infection is suspected, the medical provider will ususally start an antibiotic (doxycycline, unless one is allergic to it) at the initial visit, while waiting for the blood test restults to come back. If the blood test is positive for a tick-borne infection, the antibiotic will need to be continued and a full course will need to be completed. If the blood tests are negative for any tick-borne infection, the antibiotic will be stopped.

## PREVENTION OF TICK BITES:

- The best way to minimize tick bites is to minimize exposure to ticks. Here are some suggestions on how to do that:
  - If possible, stay away from wooded areas, tall grasses, and leaf litter. When walking in woods, stay on the trail.
  - Wear long-sleeved shirts, long pants, high socks, boots and baseball caps. To prevent ticks from crawling under clothing, tuck the long pants into the socks and the shirt into the pants.
  - Use insect repellant that contains DEET (30% or less); it is safe to spray this on clothing as well as skin. . DEET is effective in repelling ticks.
  - After being outside, everyone needs to be checked for ticks everywhere on the body, including the scalp (which can be somewhat tedious). If any ticks are found, remove them and discard them in a safe place.
  - Any clothing that had been worn outside in tick infested areas can be treated by putting it in a dryer on high heat for 20-30 minutes.

# BEES, WASP AND HORNET STINGS

## CAUSES:
- Children may be stung almost anywhere on the body - face and head, neck, arms, legs, and trunk.

## SYMPTOMS:
- A local area of redness, swelling and warmth at the site of the sting are the most common reactions to an insect sting.
- Infrequently, hives, swelling of lips and tongue, shortness of breath, vomiting and/or diarrhea may occur. **If any of these symptoms develop in your child, call 911. If available, give Benadryl® immediately.** (See dosage chart in appendix). **This is a medical emergency.**

## WHAT TO DO AT HOME:
- Give your child a dose of Benadryl® soon after the sting; it can be repeated every 4 hours as long as there is any itching.
- Apply a cool compress to the sting site – this will help reduce swelling.
- Observe for any other symptoms listed above over the next 4-6 hours.
- Swelling can occur despite cool compresses occasionally; in fact, swelling can be worse in the next one to two days following the sting than on the initial day. Continue cool compresses and Benadryl®.

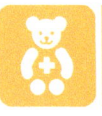

### WHEN TO CONTACT YOUR CHILD'S HEALTHCARE PROVIDER
- **When the degree of swelling at the site of the sting is uncomfortable.**

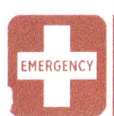

## WHEN TO CALL 911 or GO TO THE EMERGENCY ROOM

- **If any of the following symptoms are present shortly after the sting: hives, swelling of lip/tongue, shortness of breath, vomiting, diarrhea.**

## DIAGNOSIS AND TREATMENT:

- Your child's medical provider or the Emergency Room will perform a physical examination.
- Depending on the allergic symptoms present and their severity, the provider may order adrenaline (epinephrine) in the form of an injection, antihistamines IV and oral or injected steroids. A child with a significan allergic reaction to an insect sting should be prescribed an EpiPen® (ephinephrine) to have at all times in case of another sting/bite in the future.
- If seen in the Emergency Room for a significan allergic reaction, your child should follow up with his own medical provider soon. Children who have had a significant allergic reaction to an insect sting are prescribed an Epipen® (injectable epinephrine) to be used if they are inadvertently stung again in the future. Getting an INSECT STING ALLERGY PLAN in place is important for the proper management of any future insect stings. This outlines exactly what should be done in the case of another sting. This plan should be shared with anyone who will have the child under their care and guidance (relatives, school, babysitter). A referral to an allergist would be recommended as well to see if your child would be a candidate for desensitization allergy injections (similar to allergy shots).

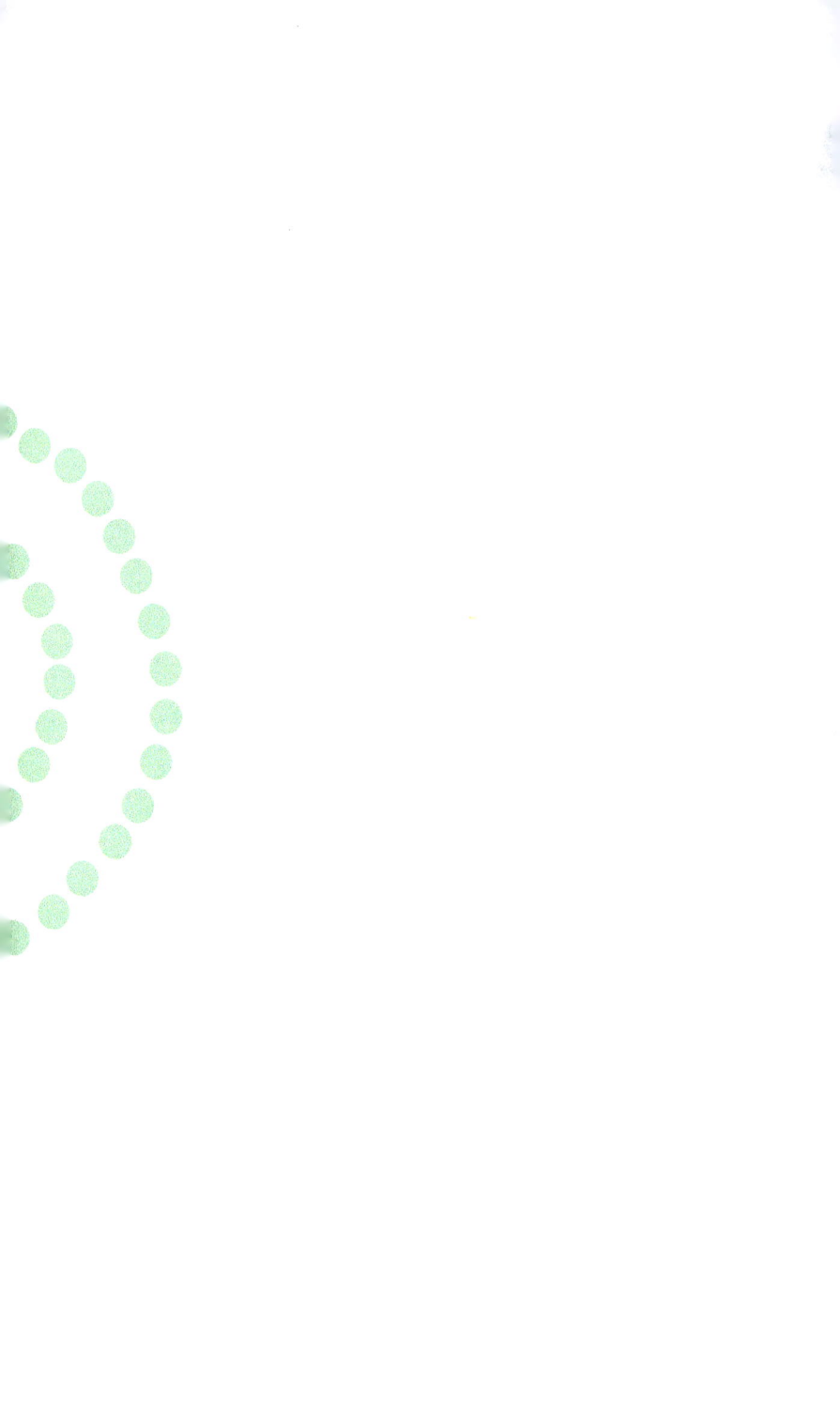

# CHAPTER 12
# MISCELLANEOUS

# FEVER

> A very common problem that children of all ages experience from time to time during infancy, toddler years, and childhood years. Adolescents experience fever less often than younger age groups.

## CAUSES:

- INFECTION is the most common cause of fever in children. The most common type of infections are caused by viruses, followed by bacterial infections, and then fungal infections.
- After infection, INFLAMMATION is the next most common cause of fever in children. Inflammation occurs when the immune system is in "overdrive" — as in rheumatoid arthritis, lupus, or post-viral infection.
- Some forms of cancer will present with prolonged fever.
- Immunizations will sometimes cause fever a day or two after a child receives the vaccine; this is a less common reason now than in the past.
- Teething may cause a low grade fever.

## SYMPTOMS:

- Definition of an elevated body temperature is:

    - 100.4 degrees F (38 degrees C) when taken rectally.
    - 99.5 degrees F (37.5 degrees C) when taken orally.

- Your child may act like he/she does not feel well.
- Your child may act normal.
- Your child's heart rate will be elevated when fever is present.
- Your child's respiratory rate will be increased when fever is present.

## HOW TO TREAT AT HOME:

- Treat the fever with acetominophen (Tylenol®) or ibuprofen (Motrin®, Advil®) if your child:
    - Is still playing;
    - Is eating and drinking OK
    - Is alert, smiling and/or talking to you;
    - Has normal skin color
    - Looks OK when the temperature is normal or close to normal
- Dress the child in light weight clothes – do not bundle up your child, even if he/she is having chills.
- Give your child a lukewarm to warm bath (as long the temperature of the water is a little cooler than your child, it will help lower the body temperature);
- <u>Do not give a rubbing alcohol bath – this is no longer recommended and is actually dangerous.</u>
- <u>Never use ice or a cold water bath to treat a fever.</u>
- Encourage your child to drink liquids (preferably cool liquids)
- SEE DOSAGE CHART FOR MEDICATIONS THAT TREAT FEVER IN APPENDIX.

## Miscellaneous

**EMERGENCY**

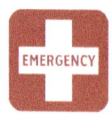

**WHEN TO CALL YOUR CHILD'S MEDICAL PROVIDER FOR AN URGENT APPOINTMENT OR GO TO THE EMERGENCY ROOM IF YOU CANNOT CONTACT YOUR PROVIDER**

- **The child is 2 months of age or less with a rectal temp of 100.4 degrees F or greater.**
- **There is a rash or new bruises present with the fever.**
- **The child cannot be awakened easily.**
- **The child is complaining of a very bad headache.**
- **The child has a stiff neck.**
- **The child is refusing to move an extremity.**
- **The child has a seizure.**
- **The child is confused.**
- **The child is not eating or drinking at all.**
- **The child is having shortness of breath.**
- **The child has recently traveled to another country.**
- **The child has a weakened immune system.**
- **If your child has a serious health condition such as diabetes, heart disease, sickle cell disease.**
- **IF ANY OF THE ABOVE CONDITIONS ARE PRESENT, CONTACT YOUR CHILD'S MEDICAL PROVIDER IMMEDIATELY OR GO TO THE EMERGENCY ROOM.**

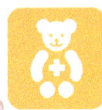

### WHEN TO CONTACT YOUR CHILD'S HEALTHCARE PROVIDER FOR A SAME-DAY SICK APPOINTMENT

- **If there are complaints of ear pain, throat pain, vomiting or significant cough.**
- **If the fever is greater than 102 degrees F in a 2-12 month-old.**
- **If the fever has been present for greater than 24-48 hours in a less than 2 year old child.**
- **If the fever has been present for greater that 48-72 hours in a child older than 2 years of age.**
- **If your child has a low grade fever for greater than 5 days.**
- **If you have any concerns.**

## DIAGNOSIS AND TREATMENT:

- After taking a history, the medical provider will always do a physical exam to look for obvious reasons for the fever.
- Sometimes, lab tests (either done in the office or at a lab) will be performed.
- Sometimes, xrays may be needed to help with the work up.
- The treatment recommended will be dependent on the cause of the fever. AN ANTIBIOTIC IS NOT NECESSARY/INDICATED IN ALL CASES OF FEVER.

## IMPORTANT:

- In and of itself, fever is not a dangerous thing; but it can occasionally be part of a serious problem.
- A fever is what the body uses to help fight infections.
- The temperature control center in the brain will not allow a temperature to become so elevated as to cause brain injury.

# HOW TO TAKE A TEMPERATURE:

NOTE:
- RECTAL temperatures are most accurate.
- FOREHEAD temperatures are next most accurate.
- ORAL and EAR temperatures are accurate if done properly.
- AXILLARY (armpit) are least accurate.

- In children under 4 months of age, taking a rectal temperature is recommended. Apply some Vaseline or other lubricant to the end of the thermometer and insert the tip into the rectum about one half inch. This is best done with the infant on their stomach or side. Using your hand, squeeze the buttocks together which will then hold the thermometer easily in place. Leave the thermometer in until it beeps. (Make sure to clean off the temperature probe after using).

- A forehead touch probe can be used on any age infant (older than 4 months) or a child. Run the probe (that is in direct contact with the skin) from the middle of the forehead over to in front of the ear. Stop when you reach the hairline. The temperature will be displayed immediately.

- An ear temperature is taken by pulling the ear upward and backward and aiming the ear probe between the opposite eye and ear. The temperature will be displayed in about 2 seconds. This test is accurate in children older than 6 months of age. (Make sure that the child has been inside for at least 15 minutes before taking an ear temperature).

- An oral temperature can be taken in a cooperative child older than 4 years of age. The tip of the thermometer needs to be placed under the side of the tongue and the mouth needs to remain shut for the test to be accurate. One needs to wait about 30 minutes after a drink for the temperature to reflect the true body temperature. Hold the thermometer in the mouth until it beeps – about 10 seconds.

- It is not recommended to take an axillary temperature.

# NAIL BITING

> Nail biting is a common and frustrating habit for many children, teens, and parents. Roughly half of all children bite their nails and it is more common in boys than girls after the age of 10.

## CAUSES:

- Nails may not be well-trimmed.
- Children may see other people do it.
- Children may do it to give their brain some extra stimulation.
- Children may do it to deal with stress and anxiety.

## THERE ARE A FEW THINGS THAT PARENTS CAN DO TO HELP WITH NAIL BITING:

- REPLACEMENT BEHAVIOR:
  - Distract your child when you see them biting their nails. encourage them to do an activity for you.
  - Teach a more tolerable behavior (playing with some object – squeezing a ball).
  - Have them do something annoying before they are allowed to bite their nails (wiggle fingers for 30 seconds) They might just get annoyed enough to stop!
  - Have them sit on their hands or do arm movements when you see them biting their nails.

- **INCREASE AWARENESS OF BITING:**

  - Saying "stop" or "knock it off" can increase stress for you and your child which might actually make nail biting worse.
  Instead, come up with a code word or secret sign (ie, tugging on your ear) to let your child know when they are biting. Your child can also share this word or sign with friends, teachers, coaches, etc. so that they can help as well.

- **BUILD AND MAINTAIN MOTIVATION:**

  - Use a reward system for your child.
  - Set a timer and give your child one point if they are able to go the whole time without biting.
  They can then use the points accumulated overtime to "buy" a reward.

# TICS

- Short lasting sudden movements, normally involving the eyelids, face, neck and shoulder that spontaneously occur and are repetitive (motor tics).
- Occur during otherwise normal behavior; a child cannot control tics (just like we cannot control hiccups).
- There are vocal tics as well – sudden grunts, short cough and throat clearing are some examples.
- Age of onset is 6-7 years of age.
- Usually tics last less than one year; some children have tics for longer periods of time but they usually disappear in the teenage years.
- More common in boys (3:1 compared with girls); approximately 20 % of all children have a tic at sometime.
- No treatment is necessary as long as tics remain simple (just one repetitive movement) and the tics do not bother the person who has them, they do not interfere with school work, or become a social impairment.
- TOURETTE'S SYNDROME is the combination of both motor and vocal tics that have lasted for at least one year. Normally it is diagnosed by a neurologist with the given history and physical exam.
There is not a test (blood or imaging) that makes the diagnosis. Tourette's is not curable but it can be treated to minimize the tics.

## WHAT TO DO:

- As long as tics remain simple and do not interfere with activities of daily living, the child can be observed; it should be mentioned at your child's yearly physical.
- If the tic, even though simple, starts to interfere with school work or social interactions, make an appointment to see your child's medical provider.
- If there is a combination of motor and vocal tics that are present for greater than 3 months, make an appointment with your child's medical provider. Referral to a pediatric neurologist may be recommended.
- If other abnormal behaviors start to occur in addition to the tics, contact your child's provider.

## NOTE:

- TICS and Tourette's syndrome can be associated with other disorders such as Attention Deficit Disorder, anxiety, Oppositional Defiant Disorder or Obsessive Compulsive Disorder.

# CAR SEAT INFO GUIDE

## IMPORTANT POINTS:

CAR SEAT TYPES ARE DEPENDENT ON:
- The age of the child.
- The size of the child.
- The developmental stage of the child.

CAR SEATS CAN BE ATTACHED TO A CAR SEAT BY EITHER:
- LATCH (Lower Anchors and Tethers for Children) system. This is present in all vehicles made after September 2002.
- Seat belts.

- It is important to read both the car owner's manual as well as the car seat manual before installing the car seat.
- Children less than 13 years of age need to sit in the back seat.
- All infants and toddlers should ride in REAR FACING only car seats until they max out the height and weight limits of the car seat; then they may go to a CONVERTIBLE REAR FACING car seat.
- A recline feature of a car seat should be considered for a child who has a disability associated with weak neck muscles.
- Dress the child appropriately for sitting in the car seat; bulky clothing should be removed prior to strapping the child in. If necessary a blanket can be thrown over the child after he or she has been strapped in for needed warmth.
- It is OK for a rear-facing child's feet to touch the seat; he or she will not be uncomfortable.

# TYPES OF CAR SEATS:

### ▸ DEPENDENT ON AGE OF CHILD:

INFANTS AND TODDLERS:
- Rear Facing only.
- Convertible seat.
- All-in-one.

TODDLERS AND PRESCHOOLERS:
- Convertible seat.
- Combination seat.

SCHOOL AGE CHILD:
- Combination seat.
- Belt positioning booster.

OLDER CHILD:
- Seat belts.

### ▸ CAR SEAT FEATURES:

REAR FACING ONLY:
This type of seat typically has a handle attached to it for easy carrying of the infant in the car seat.

- Make sure to check your car seat's limitations for height and weight - this is noted on the label attached to the car seat.
- Maximum child weight ranges are normally 22 to 35 lbs.
- Maximum child length ranges are 26 to 35 inches.
- A rear facing car seat should never be placed in the front seat for traveling purposes.

## Miscellaneous

CONVERTIBLE CAR SEAT:
- Can be rear facing and then converted to a forward facing car seat when the rear facing height and weight limits have been reached.
- Typically convertible car seats have higher rear facing height and weight limits (for example up to 35 to 40 lbs and 36 inches).
- Has a 5 point harness; the harness should be tight over the shoulders and the chest clip even with the armpits and located in the center of the chest.
- When using a convertible car seat in the rear facing position the shoulder straps need to be at or just below the height of the child's shoulders.
- When using a convertible car seat in the forward-facing position the shoulder straps need to be just above or at the height of the child's shoulders.
- When using a convertible car seat make sure that the seat belt is routed through the correct path if the seat belt is the anchor.
- When using a convertible car seat that is attached via the latch system make sure that the weight of the car seat and child does not exceed the max weight for the latch. This weight limit can be found on the label of the car seat; in addition when using the latch system in a forward facing convertible car seat make sure that the top of the car seat is attached to the tether.
- Always make sure that the angle of the seat is correct.
- It is important for a child to ride in a 5-point harness until the age of 4 or 40 pounds.
- A child has outgrown a convertible car seat when:
    - Maximum height and weight limits of the car seat have been reached.
    - The child's shoulders are higher than the straps.
    - The top of the child's ears are at the top of the seat.

ALL-IN-ONE CAR SEAT:
- Can be used for rear facing, forward facing and seat belt positioning booster car seats options.
- All the above key points under convertible car seat are relevant for this type of car seat.

COMBINATION CAR SEAT:
- A combination seat with harness is suitable for forward facing with a maximum child weight of 40 to 65 lbs.
- A combination seat (without the harness) is suitable for forward facing with a maximum child weight of 100 to 120 lbs (using the seat belt shoulder strap.

BOOSTER SEATS:
- Is for the child who has outgrown the forward facing car seat limits of height and weight.
- Should be used until the child reaches 45 inches and 10 to 12 years of age.
- Booster seats allow the seat belt to fit properly over the front of the child.
- High back and backless booster seats are held in place with seatbelts only.

# WHEN IS A CHILD OLD ENOUGH TO USE JUST A SEAT BELT:

▸ When sitting in a car's seat, the child's legs can bend at 90° over the front of the seat.

# RE-USING A CAR SEAT AFTER AN ACCIDENT :

▸ After an accident, a car seat can continue to be used if 1) the vehicle can be driven off, 2) the car door next to the car seat is not damaged, 3) airbags did not deploy and 4) no damage to the car seat can be seen.

# FIRST AID

## CHAPTER 13

# CHOKING

> If you feel that your child has swallowed something and is now choking as evidenced by them holding their throat, having a scared look on their face, or an inability to cry or speak, do the following:

- **Cry for help. Dial 911.**
- **If your child is an infant**, place the child upside down in your hand (the chest in contact with your hand) with the upper part of the body slanting downward). Give several good blows with your hand in the middle of the back just below the shoulder blades. Periodically check the mouth for any object; do not swipe your finger around in the mouth – you may push the object down further.
- **If your child is too big for the above technique**, place him/her face down on your lap with the chest in contact with your legs. Give several sharp blows with your hand in the mid back region just below the shoulder blades. Periodically, check the mouth for an object.
- **If the above technique is not successful**, stand your child up with his/her back to you. Reaching around to the front of your child with your hand and arms, clench your hands and place them about halfway between your child's waist and lower edge of the rib cage.
- Give a few rapid thursts upward towards the rib cage with the idea that you are forcing air up the windpipe to hopefully dislodge the foreign object.
- **If you are still unsuccessful with the above methods**, start mouth to mouth resuscitation until EMS arrives.

- Keep in mind that choking is not gagging; gagging is not an emergency whereas choking is.

# INGESTIONS

## "MY CHILD SWALLOWED SOMETHING!"

- Children explore objects by putting them in their mouth; then, just like that, they swallow the object!
- Common items swallowed include coins and plastic beads. Don't forget medicines! Toddlers are the most common age group to put everything in their mouths.
- Objects that are dime and nickel sized move easily down the esophagus, through the stomach and out into the intestines where they easily travel and exit through the rectum. Normally, there is no pain associated with a swallowed smaller coin.
- When objects are bigger and roughly the size of a quarter, there is a chance that they could become stuck in the esophagus. This will produce pain or discomfort – grabbing the chest area and acting as if one is in pain may be how your toddler who does not yet talk gives you the clue that something is wrong.
- If a larger object makes it down the esophagus without getting stuck, it may have difficulty getting out of the stomach or could lead to a blockage somewhere in the intestine. Symptoms of these possibilities would potentially be vomiting or abdominal pain (sometimes significant).
- In addition to objects, children also explore liquids in container (cleaning solutions, for example), and cleaning pods for dishwashers and clothing, and anything else they can find in containers that they should not find (scouring powders, mice control products – for example). Many of these items have the potential to have toxic ingredients. Symptoms that a child may exhibit after ingestion of such products may include: throat pain, drooling, chest pain, stomach pain, lethargy or unconsciousness.

## WHAT TO DO AT HOME:

- If you are certain that what your child swallowed was a small coin or small plastic object and there is no noticeable pain or discomfort, you can observe your child at home. Checking stools over the next several days looking for the object is indicated. On an average, it takes 2 – 7 days for a small coin to pass.
- **If you feel that your child swallowed a medicine or some other liquid substance, call Poison Control immediately. Before you call, have the name of the medication/liquid available as well as potentially how much your child may have taken.**

# POISON CONTROL NUMBER: 800-222-1222

## WHEN TO CALL YOUR CHILD'S PROVIDER OR GO TO THE E.R.

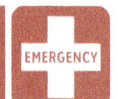

- **If you suspect that your child swallowed any of the following, go to the Emergency Room promptly: magnets, button batteries, nails, straight pins and safety pins, pieces of broken glass, or other sharp objects**
- **If your child is drooling, acting in pain, holding the chest, vomiting, or having any difficulty with breathing, go to the Emergency Room promptly.**
- **DO NOT GIVE ANY FOOD OR LIQUID IN THESE CIRCUMSTANCES!**
  **The only exception to this is in the situation of a swallowed button battery – and if your child is older than one year. Give 2 teaspoons of honey every 10 minutes until arriving at the hospital – this should help protect the lining of the esophagus from battery injury.**

## WHAT WILL BE DONE AT THE EMERGENCY ROOM/HOSPITAL:

- If the swallowed object appears to be in the esophagus and is not moving, it can be removed with instruments (via endoscopy) by a pediatric gastroenterologist.
- If the object appears to be moving and your child is comfortable, the provider will probably choose to observe and wait for passage of the object.
- If more than one magnet has been swallowed, there is a strong possibility that your child will require surgery to remove the magnets. Magnets can lead to serious damage and/or perforation of the intestinal wall if not removed promptly.
- If a button battery has been swallowed by your child it will need to be removed via endoscopy from the esophagus or stomach as soon as possible.
- If an ingestion of a medicine or toxic liquid/solid product has occurred, treatment will be dependent on what was ingested. There are specific protocols using IV fluids, certain medications, and sometimes hospitalization that has to occur.

## IMPORTANT POINTS:

- Prevention is paramount to children swallowing objects.
- Avoid having any toys that contain magnets or batteries that children can find.
- Avoid having loose change laying around.
- Avoid small toys and toys that have small parts that potentially can be swallowed by toddlers.
- Maintain clean floors – with toddlers closer to the floor than adults, they can easily find things that have fallen off tables and counter space.
- Keep all household cleaning products in a child proof cabinet or closet. Insect and mice control products should be kept in a similar location.

## IMPORTANT POINTS:

- Avoid giving younger children peanuts, small hard candy, and popcorn – these are easy foods to choke on.
- Please keep all medicines out of reach and exploration by children. <u>THIS ALSO INCLUDES ALL PRODUCTS THAT HAVE MARIJUANA AS AN INGREDIENT.</u>

## HOUSEHOLD ITEMS THAT SHOULD BE INACCESSIBLE TO CHLDREN — ESPECIALLY YOUNGER CHILDREN:

- Button batteries (many toys have these).
- Magnets (these come in ALL sizes and shapes).
- Safety pins (including open ones) and straight pins.
- Razor blades.
- Coins.
- Tiny plastic toys and children's game pieces.
- Marbles.
- Small plastic building blocks.
- Medicines, supplements, and any type of drug – including marijuana-containing foods and candies.
- Balloons ----- the danger with a balloon (one that is blown up) is the possibility that if a child would bite into one, the balloon could explode into the mouth and obstruct the child's airway.
- Cleaning solvents and paint thinners.
- Toilet bowl cleaners.
- Drano/drain cleaners.
- Dishwasher and laundry detergent/pods.
- Scouring powders.
- Insect/mice control products.
- Baby powders (inhalation of these can cause a serious lung injury).

# APPENDIX

# VITAL SIGNS: What is normal?

### HEART RATE

| AGE | BEATS PER MINUTE |
|---|---|
| 0 - 7 days | 100-180 |
| 1 - 3 weeks | 100-180 |
| 1 - 6 months | 90-180 |
| 6 - 12 months | 90-160 |
| 1 - 3 years | 90-150 |
| 4 - 5 years | 70-140 |
| 6 - 8 years | 60-120 |
| 9 - 11 years | 60-110 |
| 12 - 16 years | 60-110 |
| 16 years | 60-100 |

### RESPIRATORY RATE

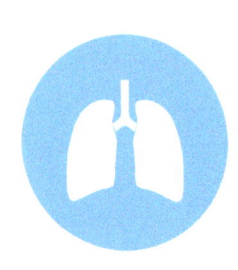

| AGE | BREATHS PER MINUTE |
|---|---|
| 0 - 1 year | 24-38 |
| 1 - 3 years | 22-30 |
| 4 - 6 years | 20-24 |
| 7 - 9 years | 18-24 |
| 10 - 14 years | 16-22 |
| 14 - 18 years | 14-20 |

### TEMPERATURE

- Can range from 97.9 to 100.4 degrees Fahrenheit as measured rectally.
- Can range from 96.9 to 99.5 degrees Fahrenheit as measured by ear, temporal or oral methods.

# TEMPERATURE CONVERSION CHART:

| Fahrenheit (°F) | Celsius (°C) |
|---|---|
| 98.6 | 37.0 |
| 99.0 | 37.2 |
| 99.5 | 37.5 |
| 100.0 | 37.8 |
| 100.4 | 38.0 |
| 101.0 | 38.3 |
| 101.3 | 38.5 |
| 102.0 | 38.9 |
| 102.2 | 39.0 |
| 103.0 | 39.4 |
| 104.0 | 40.0 |
| 105.0 | 40.5 |
| 106.0 | 41.0 |

# RECOMMENDED MEDICATIONS TO HAVE IN YOUR MEDICINE CABINET FOR CHILDREN:

- **Acetaminophen - Brand name: Tylenol®**
- **Ibuprofen - Brand name: Advil®, Motrin®**
- **Diphenhydramine - Brand name: Benadryl®**
- **Ear pain drops: 4% lidocaine**
- **Hydrocortisone 1% cream**
- **Triple antibiotic ointment: Cortisporin®, Neosporin® etc.**
- **Anti-bacterial soap**
- **Petroleum jelly - Brand name: Vaseline®**
- **Zinc oxide**

# MEDICATIONS FOR TREATING FEVER AND PAIN:

▸ **ACETAMINOPHEN/PARACETAMOL - Brand name: TYLENOL®**

| Weight | Age | Infant drops (160 mg/5mL) | Children's liquid (160 mg/5mL) | Children's chewable tablets (160 mg) |
|---|---|---|---|---|
| 6-11 lbs | 0-6 months | 1.25 mL | 1.25 mL | — |
| 12-17 lbs | 6-11 months | 2.5 mL | 2.5 mL | — |
| 18-23 lbs | 12-23 months | 3.75 mL | 3.75 mL | — |
| 24-35 lbs | 2-3 years | 5 mL | 5 mL | 1 tablet |
| 36-47 lbs | 4-5 years | 7.5 mL | 7.5 mL | 1.5 tablets |
| 48-59 lbs | 6-8 years | — | 10 mL | 2 tablets |
| 60-71 lbs | 9-10 yrs. | — | 12.5 mL | 2.5 tablets |
| 72-95 lbs | 11 years | — | 15 mL | 3 tablets |

Note : infant acetaminophen and children's acetaminophen suspension are the same concentration; it is not necessary to purchase intant drops for infants.

Dosing: acetaminophen may be given every 4 - 6 hours as needed (no more than 5 doses per day).

## Appendix

▸ **IBUPROFEN - Brand name: ADVIL®, MOTRIN®**

| Weight | Age | Infant's Drops 50 mg/1.25 mL | Children's Liquid 100 mg/5 mL | Children's tablets 100 mg | Adult tablets 200 mg |
|---|---|---|---|---|---|
| 0-11 lbs | 0-5 months | — | — | — | — |
| 12-17 lbs | 6-11 months | 1.25 mL | 2.5 mL | — | — |
| 18-23 lbs | 12-23-months | 1.875 mL | 4 mL | — | — |
| 24-35 lbs | 2-3 years | 2.5 mL | 5 mL | 1 tablet | — |
| 36-47 lbs | 4-5 years | 3.75 mL | 7.5 mL | 1.5 tabs. | — |
| 48-59 lbs | 6-8 years | 5 mL | 10 mL | 2 tablets | 1 tablet |
| 60-71 lbs | 9-10 years | — | 12.5 mL | 2.5 tabs. | 1 tablet |
| 72-95 lbs | 11 years | — | 15 mL | 3 tablets | 1.5 tabs. |
| 96+ lbs | 12+ years | — | 20 mL | 4 tablets | 2 tablets |

Dosing: ibuprofen may be given every 6 - 8 hours as needed. Max 4 doses.

Note: ibuprofen is not recommended for infants under 6 months.

# MEDICATIONS FOR TREATING ALLERGIES:

▸ **DIPHENHYDRAMINE - Brand name: BENADRYL®**

| Weight | Children's Liquid Suspension (12.5 mg/5 mL) | Children's Chewable Tablets (12.5 mg) | Children's Meltaway Strips (12.5 mg) |
|---|---|---|---|
| 10-16 lbs | 2.5 mL | — | — |
| 17-22 lbs | 3.75 mL | — | — |
| 22-26 lbs | 5 mL | 1 tablet | 1 meltaway |
| 27-32 lbs | 6.25 mL | 1 tablet | 1 meltaway |
| 33-37 lbs | 7.5 mL | 1 tablet | 1 meltaway |
| 38-43 lbs | 8.75 mL | 1 tablet | 1 meltaway |
| 44-54 lbs | 10 mL | 2 tablets | 2 meltaways |
| 55-65 lbs | 12.5 mL | 2 tablets | 2 Meltaways |
| 66-76 lbs | 15 mL | 3 tablets | 3 Meltaways |
| 77-87 lbs | 17.5 mL | 3 tablets | 3 Meltaways |
| 88+ lbs | 20 mL | 4 tablets | 4 Meltaways |

Diphenhydramine is indicated for children 6 months and older.

Dosing: Diphenhydramine may be given every 6 hours as needed.

- **LORATADINE - Brand name: CLARITIN®**
- **CETIRIZINE - Brand name: ZYRTEC®**

| Age | Children's Liquid (5 mg/5 mL) | Children's Chewable Tablets (5 mg) | Adults Tablets (10 mg) |
|---|---|---|---|
| 1-2 years | 2.5 mL/day | — | — |
| 2-6 years | 2.5-5 mL/day | 0.5-1 tablets per day | — |
| 6+ years | 5-10 mL/day | 1-2 tablets per day | 1 tablet per day |

Dosing is recommeded once daily.

- **FEXOFENADINE - Brand name: ALLEGRA®**

| Age | Children's Liquid (30 mg/5 mL) | Adult Tablets (60 mg) | Adults Tablets (180 mg) |
|---|---|---|---|
| 2-12 years | 5 mL twice/daily | — | — |
| 12+ years | 10 mL twice/daily | 1 tablet twice/daily | 1 tablet ONCE/daily |

Dosing is recommeded every 12 hours.

# MEDICATIONS FOR TREATING ACID REFLUX:

▸ **ALUMINUM/MAGNESIUM HYDROXIDE - Brand name: MAALOX®**

| Age | MaaLox® Regular Strength |
|---|---|
| 6-12 years | 5-10 mL every 3-6 hours |
| 12+ years | 10-30 mL every 3-6 hours |

Consult your child's healthcare provider for further advice after 3 doses.

# MEDICATIONS FOR CONSTIPATION:

## STOOL SOFTENERS — work by drawing more water into stool.

- **DOCUSATE SODIUM (Pedia-Lax®)**
  Dosage:
  - 2-5 years of age: 1-3 chewable tablets daily;
  - 6-11 years of age: 3-6 chewable tablets daily; (drink 8 oz. of liquid with each dose).
  
  OR
  - 2-5 years of age: 1 tablespoon daily;
  - 6-11 years of age: 3 tablespoons daily.
  (drink 8 oz. of liquid with each dose).

DO NOT GIVE FOR MORE THAN 3 CONSECUTIVE DAYS WITHOUT SPEAKING WITH YOUR CHILD'S PROVIDER.

## STIMULANT LAXATIVES — work by stimulating the muscles of the colon to push the stool along.

- **SENNA (Sennakot®)**
  Dosage for chewable tablets:
  - 6-11 years: 1 tablet, 1-2 doses/day;
  - 12 years and older: 2 tablets, 1-2 doses/day.
  
  Dosage for oral liquid:
  - 2-6 years of age: 2.5-3.75 mL per day;
  - 6-11 years of age: 5-7.5 mL per day;
  - 12 years and older: 10-15 mL per day.

- **BISACODYL (Dulcolax®)**
  Dosage for chewable tablets:
  - 3-10 years of age: 5 mg daily (1 tablet);
  - 10 years of age: 10 mg daily (2 tablets).

DO NOT GIVE FOR MORE THAN 3 CONSECUTIVE DAYS WITHOUT SPEAKING WITH YOUR CHILD'S PROVIDER.

## OSMOTIC LAXATIVES — work by bringing more water into the intestine to help soften stools.

▸ **PolyEthyleneGlycol/PEG (Miralax®)**

| Age | Single Dose | For cleanout | For maintenance | Volume of liquid needed to mix each dose |
|---|---|---|---|---|
| 6-12 months | 1 teaspoon | 2 times/day | 1 time/day | 4 oz |
| 1-3 years | 2 teaspoons | 2-3 times/day | 1 time/day | 4 oz |
| 4-7 years | 4 teaspoons | 2-3 times/day | 1 time/day | 8 oz |
| 8+ years | 1 capful | 2-3 times/day | 1 time/day | 8 oz |

Above dosages are "starting dose" recommendations; dosage may be increased or decreased depending on consistency of stool.

The goal of a MiraLax® dose is to create SOFT stools; assess your child's stool consistency every 3 days.
- If stool not soft enough, increase dose of Miralax® by one-half;
- If stool too loose, decrease dose of MiraLax® by one-half.

Maintain MiraLax® treatment for several months to maintain soft stools - do NOT stop MiraLax® once stools get soft.

# FOODS FOR CONSTIPATION:

- **FIBER FOODS** (to help with constipation):

    - FRUITS:
      Apples with skin.
      Pears with skin.
      Peaches with skin.
      Raspberries.
      Kiwis.
      Oranges.

    - VEGETABLES:
      Broccoli, cooked.
      Carrots, cooked.
      Cauliflowers, cooked.
      Brussel sprouts.
      Corn

    - BEANS:
      Kidney beans.
      Lima beans.
      Navy beans.

    - WHOLE GRAINS:
      Whole wheat cereal.
      Bran cereal.
      Oatmeal.
      Popcorn.

    - NUTS:
      Peanut butter.
      All nuts.

# SUGGESTED DAILY WATER AND MILK INTAKE FOR INFANTS, CHILDREN, AND ADOLESCENTS:

|       | 1-2 years | 2-4 years | 4-8 years | 8-12 years | 12+ years |
|-------|-----------|-----------|-----------|------------|-----------|
| Water | 2 cups    | 2 cups    | 2-3 cups  | 5 cups     | 6 cups    |
| Milk  | 2 cups    | 2-3 cups  | 2-3 cups  | 2-3 cups   | 2-3 cups  |
| TOTAL | 4 cups    | 4-5 cups  | 5-6 cups  | 7-8 cups   | 8-9 cups  |

1 cup = 8 oz.

\* Fluid intake should be increased with increased physical activity, as well as with increased enviromental heat and humidity.

# RECIPES:

## REHYDRATING FLUIDS
— useful in vomiting and diarrhea, fever illnesses, and active sports participation.

**RECIPE #1**
- 6 teaspoons of sugar
- ½ teaspoon of salt
- 5 cups of water

Stir the mixture until the sugar and salt have dissolved.

**RECIPE #2**
- 4 cups of Gatorade G2®
- ½ teaspoon of salt

Stir the salt into the Gatorade® until the salt has dissolved.

**RECIPE #3**
- 4 cups of water
- 1 dry chicken broth cube
- 2 tablespoons sugar

Boil the water and add the chicken broth cube; allow it to dissolve. Add the salt and sugar; stir until dissolved. Make sure fluid is cool before drinking it.

## NORMAL SALINE — can be used as a nasal drop or for sinus washings

**RECIPE:**
- 2 cups of water
- 1 teaspoon of salt

Bring mixture to a boil, cover and boil for 15 minutes. Store in clean container after cooling.

# INDEX

Abdominal pain, 86
Allergic rhinitis (hay fever), 44
Appendicitis, 86
Asthma (reactive airway disease), 66
Bedwetting, 133
Bites and stings:
    animal bites, 204
    bees, wasps, hornets, 210
    mosquitos, 206
    ticks, 207
Breast buds, 71
Bronchiolitis, 61
Burns, 200
Car seat information, 223
Chalazion, 36
Chest pain, 74
Chest wall defects, 73
Choking, 228
Chondromalacia patella, 141
Conjunctivitis, 34
Constipation, 91
Coughs, 58
Croup, 59
Diarrhea: bacterial, 97
      from antibiotic, 101
      from food allergy, 102
      parasitic, 100
      viral, 94
Ear infections: middle, 25
       serous (with effusion), 28
       Swimmer's ear, 30
Epididymitis, 126
Eye scratch, 38
Fainting (syncope), 81
Fever, 214
Foot pain, 148
Fractures, 143
Functional abdominal pain, 89
Gastroesophageal reflux (acid reflux), 55, 70, 106
Growing pains, 137

Head lice, 20
Head trauma, 10
Headaches, 14
Heel pain (Sever's Disease), 142
Hip pain, 139
Hydrocoele, 128
Influenza, 49
Ingestions, 229
Inguinal hernia, female, 122
Inguinal hernia, male, 131
Injuries:
- extremities, 143
- Nursemaid's elbow, 146

Intussusception, 87
Jaw pain (temporomandibular junction pain), 24
Lacerations, scalp, 12
Medications, dosages, 237
Mononucleosis, 50
Nail biting, 219
Nosebleeds, 40
Orchitis, 126
Osgood – Schlatter Disease, 140
Overuse injuries140
Peritonsillar abscess, 53
Pinworms, 113
Pneumonia, 64
Pyloric stenosis, 111
Rashes:
- Chickenpox, 150
- Contact dermatitis, 153
- Diaper rashes, 173
- Eczema, 195
- Fifth Disease, 176
- Hand, foot, and mouth disease, 157
- Hives, 179
- Impetigo, 160
- Measles/rubella, 181
- Molluscum contagiosum, 162
- Petechiae/purpura, 184
- Pityriasis rosea, 187

Rashes:
- Poison ivy, 153
- Ringworm, 198
- Roseola, 189
- Scabies, 164
- Scarlet fever, 191
- Shingles, 167
- Viral, 193
- Warts, 170

Scrapes and cuts, 203
Scrotal pain, 126
Seizures (convulsions), 17
Sore throat causes, 48
Sprains/strains, 144
Strep throat, 51
Stye (hordeolum), 37
Tachycardia (fast heart rate), 78
Temperature, how to take, 218
Testicular torsion, 126
Tics, 221
Upper respiratory infections (colds), 42
Urinary tract infections, 116
Vaginal discharge, 120
Varicocoele, 130
Vital signs, normal values, 234
Vomiting, 103, 109, 110, 112
Vulvovaginitis, 118

# ACKNOWLEDGMENTS

I want to acknowledge the tremendous moral support of my husband, John, as well as the extra work that he has done in his semi-retired physician status to allow me the time to work on this book over the past year. In addition, similar gratitude goes to our two children, Colleen and J.C.

The other incredibly special and major contributor to this book due kudos is our "Italian daughter", Cristina; it is her design and layout that brought this book to life.

Lastly, I would be amiss if I did not acknowledge my dedicated office staff, fellow providers, and thousands of patients over the past 40+ years; without their support and trust in me, my very gratifying career in pediatrics would not be where it is today. And the desire to write this book would not have surfaced.